NURSING EVALUATION:
THE PROBLEM
AND THE PROCESS
The Critical Incident Technique

NURSING EVALUATION:
THE PROBLEM
AND THE PROCESS
The Critical Incident Technique

GRACE FIVARS

ASSISTANT TO THE DIRECTOR OF RESEARCH
AMERICAN INSTITUTES FOR RESEARCH
IN THE BEHAVIORAL SCIENCES
PITTSBURGH

DORIS GOSNELL

B.S., M.Litt., R.N.

DIRECTOR OF INSERVICE EDUCATION
PRESBYTERIAN-UNIVERSITY HOSPITAL
PITTSBURGH
FORMERLY ASSOCIATE DIRECTOR
SCHOOL OF NURSING
THE WESTERN PENNSYLVANIA HOSPITAL
PITTSBURGH

THE MACMILLAN COMPANY
New York

COLLIER-MACMILLAN LIMITED
London

The W. R. Banks Library
Prairie View A. & M. College
Prairie View, Texas

TO

all who are endeavoring to achieve

excellence in nursing

Foreword

The pursuit of excellence, if it is to be more than a mere series of bursts of activity, must have as a basic directional guide the sound evaluation of performance. The authors of this book have systematically presented the application of the wisdom which has developed through efforts to evaluate performance in many fields to problems of evaluation in nursing.

The procedures which are clearly described and illustrated here should be of great value to those responsible for achieving and maintaining a high level of performance in all areas of nursing. The book is notable for the thorough treatment given to the fundamentals of evaluation procedures. This should prove a valuable aid since the effective use of evaluation procedures in any health agency or institution requires a full understanding of the basic assumptions and theory on which these techniques are based.

The examples and references should be of special value in making practical use of evaluation procedures in the hospital setting as well as in other activities. The authors are to be commended for a well-written, well-documented discussion of this very important aspect of nursing.

JOHN C. FLANAGAN
President
American Institutes for Research
in the Behavioral Sciences

Preface

Nursing is an art and a science. Often patient progress depends on the quality of care and the knowledge, skills, and abilities of the nurse. Because of the many implications for human welfare, it is mandatory that nursing personnel achieve and maintain a high quality of performance whenever and wherever patient care is offered.

The fundamental purpose of this book is to present information about an empirical method for evaluating nursing behavior. Recent actions by national agencies in establishing standards for nursing services have lent impetus to the search for appropriate measures for evaluating nursing care. Procedures for measuring educational outcomes have been adapted from other fields, but these assess academic achievement only; they do not cover performance in clinical areas. Until recently there were no objective procedures for evaluating nursing behavior.

A major portion of this book is concerned with establishing broad, over-all institutional objectives; the development of curriculums and course content consistent with these objectives; and the selection of learning experiences designed to meet educational needs. This information should prove useful to committees on objectives in schools of nursing and to those responsible for nursing service in various health agencies. No attempt is made to set forth rigid rules for developing objectives in specific institutions—this remains the responsibility of each individual organization. The aim is to assist in creating the climate for evaluation.

Throughout the book an effort is made to reinforce discussions with examples and illustrative materials which instructors, supervisors, and administrators can adapt to fit their needs. Of particular importance is a plan for a unit of instruction in a selected area that describes in detail each step

vii

from the establishment of unit objectives through all phases of teacher and student activity to the evaluation of student learning based on changes in behavior.

Later sections of the book discuss the application of the critical incident technique to the evaluation of performance in nursing. The Clinical Experience Record is presented with examples of the classification of effective and ineffective incidents of nursing behavior. Major emphasis is given to encouraging strengths and overcoming weaknesses in performance based on a review of the record.

The book contains three appendixes: I. Lists of critical requirements in fields related to nursing. These are intended to demonstrate the outcome of research studies aimed at identifying critical behaviors important to successful performance in specific activities. II. Lists of expected student behavior based on objectives in selected clinical areas. III. Performance descriptions of selected nursing functions and procedures. Materials for Appendixes II and III were developed on the basis of needs and requirements in a specific institution or group of institutions. They are not intended for direct application to all situations in nursing. Howeve, they should be useful as models on which to develop procedures for specific educational programs or activities for nursing service.

The book is intended primarily as a text and a reference for instructors and others interested in nursing. Educators and those responsible for nursing service administration should find it a valuable resource. It should also serve as a reference for graduate students and clinical specialists who will eventually be responsible for evaluating nursing personnel.

The authors are indebted to Dr. John C. Flanagan, President of the American Institutes for Research, for permitting them to use materials on the critical incident technique which he developed and for allowing them to draw heavily on the rich resources of the research conducted by personnel of the Institutes. A word of grateful appreciation—

To Dr. Robert M. Gagné for the many valuable suggestions he offered. Much of the information on curriculum development and learning experiences was derived from his research and writings.

To Dr. and Mrs. Robert Fitzpatrick for their intensive review of the manuscript and their assistance on sections relating to evaluation and testing.

To Mrs. Angeline Marchese Jacobs, R.N., for her original contributions to the research to develop the Clinical Experience Record and for her extensive work in providing performance descriptions of specific nursing procedures. Mrs. Jacobs provided technical assistance both as a psychologist and as a nurse.

To Mr. Daryl G. Nichols for his pinpoint review of the manuscript through many stages of development. He was particularly gracious in assisting on sections concerned with task analysis and testing.

To Miss Mary Edwards, R.N., who reviewed the technical content of the book on the basis of her years of experience in nursing and nursing education.

To Dr. Paul P. Mok for a marvelous moment of insight which resulted in the final synthesis of the manuscript.

To Mr. David H. Elder for his excellent artwork, to Mrs. Margaret L. Lere and Miss Janet R. Shaw for typing the manuscript, and to Miss Jean Cotter for helping with final preparation of the materials.

To the many authors and authorities in the fields of education, psychology, and nursing who were so generous in permitting the use of citations and quotations from their writings and reports of research.

To Mr. Henry Van Swearingen, Editor in the College and Professional Division of The Macmillan Company, for his fine editorial assistance and guidance in the preparation of the book for publication.

To the nurses in many hospitals and schools of nursing in Pittsburgh who participated in the collection of the original data for the study which led to the development of the Clinical Experience Record for evaluating nursing performance.

And finally, to our families and friends for their encouragement and moral support through the long, hot summer, and the cold, dreary winter of the year we wrote this book.

G. F.
D. G.

Contents

NURSING EVALUATION:
THE PROBLEM
AND THE PROCESS
The Critical Incident Technique

Critical Incident

There was an explosion at a local industrial plant, and the emergency room of the hospital was advised that six victims were being brought in. Miss North, a professional nursing student, was assigned to the emergency room to gain experience in the activities there. She did not know what type of explosion had occurred, however, she prepared emergency tracheostomy trays, burn dressing trays, intravenous fluids, extra blankets, and extra resuscitating equipment. She also checked the supply of emergency drugs in the medicine cupboard. She notified the supervisor immediately.

This is an effective critical incident. Although this was Miss North's first experience on the emergency room, she was quick to prepare for a minor disaster by having extra supplies and equipment in readiness for treatment of the victims. She did not rely solely on the standing orders for routine emergencies.

Chapter 1
Why Study
Nursing Behavior?

Modern nursing is entering its second century of service. Now is the time to look at present practice and plan for the future. What direction will nursing take in the next ten or twenty years? How can we use what we have learned during the past few decades? Significant changes have taken place and have had an important impact on nursing and nursing practice: changes in technology, in medical science, in standards of living, in attitudes about mental and physical health, and most importantly, in public support of research to amplify nursing resources. How can we prepare to cope with the changes and the new demands?

There is a growing awareness that nursing can make important contributions to our capability to improve and maintain mental health and physical well-being, not only in the hospital environment but in the community as well. The expanding responsibilities of nursing indicate that we should study the profession and the people in it. The development of better educational facilities and better methods for maintaining professional standards can do much to improve the effectiveness of nursing care.

Why the concern about increasing the quality of nursing and nursing care? Tyler identified several important reasons:* (1) the tremendous increase in population causes health needs to multiply proportionately;

* Ralph W. Tyler. "Changing Horizons in Nursing Education," *New Dimensions of Learning in a Free Society*, University of Pittsburgh Press, 1958, p. 177.

(2) a greater percentage of people today seek nursing service because they now enjoy the protection and benefits of prepaid hospital insurance and medical care plans; and (3) there is a marked increase in the construction of hospital facilities both public and private that make the benefits of nursing care more accessible to more people.

What are the implications of these growing demands? The accelerated requirements indicate first of all the need for a critical review of the educational programs that prepare nurses to enter the profession. What can we do to improve the quality of education in schools of nursing? Tyler describes some "changing horizons" toward which we should strive:*

1. A *science of nursing care should be developed* emphasizing the teaching of relevant principles in the basic biological sciences as they apply to nursing.
2. *Educational programs should be improved* consistent with the standards of the profession.†
3. *Schools of nursing beyond the diploma level should be developed.*
4. *The field of nursing service should be more fully developed* not only in the hospital setting but in other health agencies as well.
5. *The health team should be expanded* to meet increasing community health needs.
6. *Nursing should assume a greater share of responsibility in helping to shape social policy.*

These goals should give greater dimension to nursing. To meet the challenges, much thought and effort must be devoted to expanding, developing, and improving nursing education at all levels. We need to start by stepping up efforts to attract more young people to the profession.

In 1963 a report of the Surgeon General's Consultant Group on Nursing‡ indicated that by 1970 the nation will need 850,000 nurses. Can we bring about an increase of more than 50 per cent in the enrollment in schools of nursing during the next few years? If we hope to cope with anticipated requirements for nurses and nursing service in the 1970's, we must increase efforts to recruit new students.

Are schools of nursing equipped to prepare the kinds of nurses we will need? At present there are four types of educational programs that prepare students to enter nursing. These include:

* *Ibid.*, pp. 178-83.
† "Standards for Organized Nursing Services," *Am. J. Nursing*, 65:76-79, (March) 1965.
‡ *Toward Quality in Nursing Needs and Goals.* Report of the Surgeon General's Office Consultant Group on Nursing, U.S. Department of Health, Education, and Welfare, Washington, D.C., 1963, p. 54.

1. The *vocational school,* a one-year program designed to prepare students for work as practical nurses. The course is usually offered in a school or hospital, and graduates may apply for licensure to become practical nurses. Those who qualify and meet standards are granted licenses to perform certain routine functions and to assist professional nurses in administering specific kinds of care.
2. The *associate degree program* usually requires two years and is offered in a lower division level of a college or in a community or junior college. Upon completion of the course students may apply for a license and, if they qualify, should be prepared to give patient care as beginning staff nurses in hospitals and to assume a share of the responsibility along with other members of the nursing team in giving patient care.
3. The *diploma program* requires two to three years and is generally conducted in hospital schools of nursing. Graduates may apply for licensure and upon qualifying should be prepared to assist other members of the health team in planning and conducting programs for patient care. They should be capable of assuming responsibility for directing the activities of other members of the nursing team.
4. The *college* or *university program* in nursing usually requires four years. Graduates receive the baccalaureate degree and may apply for licensure. Those who qualify should be prepared to give nursing care and to interpret and demonstrate such care to others. Many college and university nursing graduates go on to take advanced education leading to careers in teaching and administrative activities in nursing or in nursing research.

HOW CAN THE EDUCATIONAL
PROGRAMS BE IMPROVED?

The Surgeon General's Consultant Group reported that mere increases in the number of admissions to these various types of nursing education programs will not be sufficient. More effort is needed:*

1. We must *clarify the objectives* of each of the various preparatory programs in nursing. At present the four programs overlap. We need to distinguish one from another.
2. *Student recruiting should be improved.* Better selection procedures are needed. If recruiting is improved, it can reduce the attrition in

* *Ibid.,* p. 56.

enrollment which often occurs when students lack the requisite aptitudes and abilities for success in nursing.

3. *The technical content of nursing programs should be increased.* It may be feasible to shorten the time required for teaching concentrated general nursing care, and to initiate additional programs that permit students to take advanced work in selected areas that prepare them to meet the growing need for nursing specialists in key fields.

4. *The general quality of instruction should be improved.* This is a constant need in education. Schools of nursing should make fuller use of new and modern instructional methods. Autoinstructional devices, programed learning techniques, teaching machines, television, audiovisual aids, and other recent innovations in education can all help to improve the quality of instruction and conceivably might even help to shorten the amount of time needed to complete certain required courses in nursing.

5. *Systematic evaluation of nursing performance should take place on a continuing basis.* Effective evaluation can provide increased opportunities for learning and for better teaching. Evaluation procedures should include the establishment of minimum standards of acceptable performance at the various educational levels. In addition we should consider periodic self-evaluation of nursing education at the local school level and of nursing practice at the national level.

These are just a few of the issues identified by Tyler and others. The resolution of these problems rests with the leaders in the field of nursing.

This book will address itself to some of these problems, in particular: increasing the effectiveness of nursing through nursing education, the identification and clarification of objectives in schools of nursing at both the school and curriculum levels, and the initiation of a new technique for evaluating nursing performance and behavior. The emphasis is on the use of the critical incident technique—a data-gathering process to expedite a critical review and analysis of the facts. Through this approach the authors hope to present some suggestions that may prove useful to educators in schools of nursing, to nursing practitioners, and to others in the field in their efforts to maintain the high standards of the profession in hospitals, industrial health clinics, rehabilitation centers, and other health agencies.

Bibliography
"Standards for Organized Nursing Services," *Am. J. Nursing,* 65:76-79, (March) 1965.
Toward Quality in Nursing Needs and Goals. Report of the Surgeon General's

Consultant Group on Nursing. U.S. Department of Health, Education, and Welfare, Washington, D.C. 1963.

Tyler, Ralph W. "Changing Horizons in Nursing Education," *New Dimensions of Learning in a Free Society*, University of Pittsburgh Press, 1958.

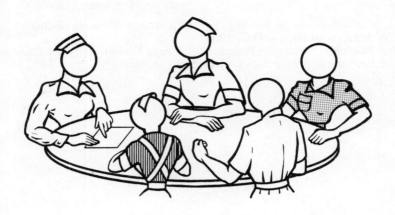

Critical Incident

Members of the nursing team were meeting to conduct the morning planning conference. Miss Gray, an advanced professional nursing student, made some notations on the nursing care plans about the anxiety she had noted in one of the preoperative patients. She also made a note about another patient who was apprehensive about the possible loss of his sight.

This is an effective critical incident. The information which Miss Gray provided voluntarily contributed to more effective patient care since other members of the nursing team would be prepared to cope with these problems after reading Miss Gray's notes on the nursing care plan. Her willingness to provide vital information about signs and symptoms of patients was evidence of good interaction with fellow team members. In addition, noting important signs and symptoms and relaying this information lead to improved patient care.

Chapter 2
The Critical Incident
Approach to
Problems in Nursing

Think of the last time you observed a nurse do something that you thought was especially effective in contributing to patient care.

What led up to the situation?

Exactly what did the nurse do?

Why do you feel it was particularly effective?

Interviewers asked these questions when the critical incident technique was used to collect information about nursing behavior. The main idea was to gather facts about nursing care to make an intensive study of nursing behavior.*

WHERE DID THE TECHNIQUE ORIGINATE?

During World War II there was urgent need to select, classify, and train thousands of recruits in a minimum amount of time.† The Air Force needed aircrewmen to man their planes. Intensive studies were conducted to find out why some men could learn to fly while others could not. What kinds of men could be trained to become pilots? Why would some men make better navigators and bombardiers? Why were some bombing missions failures? These were difficult problems. To solve them the researchers needed to collect a great deal of information.

* William A. Gorham, Stanley Lichtenstein, and Angeline C. Marchese. *Specific Nursing Behaviors Related to Patient Care and Improvement*, American Institutes for Research, Washington, D.C., 1959.

† John C. Flanagan. "The Aviation Psychology Program in the Army Air Forces," *Army Air Forces Aviation Psychology Program Research Report No. 1*, U.S. Government Printing Office, Washington, D.C., 1947, p. 51.

John C. Flanagan and members of the Aviation Psychology Program developed a method of intensive interviewing designed to eliminate generalizations, judgments, or opinions and to pinpoint the facts.* The researchers were not satisfied with the information collected from the written proceedings of elimination boards giving reasons why pilots "washed out" of flying school. Those records contained too many vague statements such as "lack of inherent flying ability," "unsuitable temperament," "poor judgment," or simply "lack of sufficient progress."† These were opinions, not facts.

Questionnaires were developed that asked straightforward questions and required straightforward answers:

Think of the last time you saw a pilot candidate do something that was ineffective.
What led up to the situation?
Exactly what did the man do?
Why was it ineffective?

These were the kinds of questions developed for questionnaires. They asked for answers based on actual observations by pilot instructors.

The same was true in the study to determine why certain bombing missions failed. The facts were needed. A similar type of interview was conducted with the men returning from the bombing missions.‡ They were asked why certain missions failed, what led up to the situation, and why the action was ineffective.

Other studies using the same technique identified behaviors important to the duties of pilots, navigators, and bombardiers. Once these behaviors were identified, it was possible to develop a battery of aptitude classification tests for use in screening applicants for the Air Force.§

This direct, factual approach for gathering information became known as the *critical incident technique*—a collection of information based on direct observation. Opinion, generalizations, and personal judgment are reduced to a minimum—only the facts are reported.

CAN THE CRITICAL INCIDENT
TECHNIQUE BE USED TO
SOLVE PRACTICAL PROBLEMS?

Following the research activities in the war, Flanagan and his staff generalized their findings to solutions of practical problems. Selection and classification tests were developed for various service and civilian jobs.

* Flanagan, *loc. cit.*
† Flanagan, *loc. cit.*
‡ Flanagan, *loc. cit.*
§ Flanagan, *op. cit.*, pp. 62-65.

Evaluation devices were developed for use in military activities and in education and industry.*

One of the first postwar studies was the development of procedures for evaluating Air Force officers. Preston collected more than 3000 incidents from 600 officers who provided information about their peers and subordinates. An analysis of this information resulted in the identification of 54 critical requirements for officers in the United States Air Force.† Six major areas of behavior were identified:

1. Proficiency in handling administrative details
2. Proficiency in supervising personnel
3. Proficiency in planning and directing action
4. Acceptance of organizational responsibility
5. Acceptance of personal responsibility
6. Proficiency in Duty Military Occupational Specialty

A close look at the key areas listed above indicates that they pinpoint the critical requirements for officers who supervise the activities of their men and at the same time must achieve the accomplishment of certain military assignments.

The technique was also used in a study of the critical requirements for research personnel working at various naval installations.‡ More than 2500 research workers contributed reports of incidents they observed on the people they worked with and those they supervised. An analysis of these incidents revealed more than 3400 different behaviors. These were classified into an organized framework which included eight critical areas of behavior important in conducting research.

1. Formulating problems and hypotheses
2. Planning and designing the investigation
3. Conducting the investigation
4. Interpreting research results
5. Preparing reports
6. Administering research projects
7. Accepting organizational responsibility
8. Accepting personal responsibility

In a later phase of this project a checklist was developed to evaluate the performance of research personnel using these critical behaviors.§

* American Institutes for Research. A *Report of Three Years of Experience*, American Institutes for Research, Pittsburgh, 1950.

† Harley O. Preston. *The Development of a Procedure for Evaluating Officers in the United States Air Force*, American Institutes for Research, Pittsburgh, 1948, pp. 45-51.

‡ John C. Flanagan *et al. Critical Requirements for Research Personnel*, American Institutes for Research, Pittsburgh, 1949, pp. 24-30.

§ Mary H. Weislogel. *Evaluating the Performance of Research Personnel*, American Institutes for Research, Pittsburgh, 1951.

These are just two of the many occupations in which the critical incident technique has been used to identify requirements. This same technique has been used for a variety of other purposes. For example, in addition to establishing criteria it has been used to—

Develop measures of proficiency (evaluation)
Establish training requirements (teaching)
Establish selection and classification requirements (screening)
Design jobs
Establish operating procedures
Develop equipment design
Motivate people to do a better job (studies of leadership, attitude, and motivation)
Counsel students (and for purposes of psychotherapy)

A list of some of the studies using critical incidents for various purposes is included in the bibliography at the end of this chapter.

HAS THE CRITICAL INCIDENT TECHNIQUE BEEN USED IN STUDIES OF NURSING?

The technique has been used in a variety of ways to study problems in nursing:

The Role of the Private Duty Nurse

Critical incidents and several other data-gathering procedures were used by Pumroy and Suttell to identify the role of the private duty nurse in the hospital environment in Washington, D.C.* Findings were reported in terms of (1) the private duty nurse as a professional working woman, (2) the private duty nurse in the hospital environment, (3) the human relations aspects of private duty nursing, and (4) sources of job satisfaction in private duty nursing. Several thousand incidents were collected from doctors, supervisors, head nurses, private duty nurses, and patients. Some were mailed in the form of anonymous written reports, others were collected on the basis of daily observation records, and still others were presented during structured interviews with nursing personnel. The incidents were classified into three main areas.†

1. Nonmedical (nontechnical) duties and responsibilities of the private duty nurse—the "extras" which the private duty nurse and others consider essential in patient care

* Shirley S. Pumroy and Barbara J. Suttell. *The Private Duty Nurse: Her Role in the Hospital Environment of Washington, D.C.*, American Institutes for Research, Washington, D.C., 1956.
† Pumroy and Suttell, *loc. cit.*

2. Sources of satisfaction with private duty nursing in the hospital environment
3. Sources of dissatisfaction with private duty nursing in the hospital environment

Analysis of these incidents provided much useful information about the role of the private duty nurse working in the hospital environment.

Identification of Nursing Behaviors Important to Patient Care

Gorham, Lichtenstein, and Marchese studied specific nursing behaviors related to patient care and improvement.* More than 2000 incidents were collected from 686 physicians, nursing supervisors, staff nurses, and patients in ten hospitals in the Washington, D.C. area. The incidents were categorized and organized into a behavioral classification system involving five major areas of performance:

1. Improving patient's adjustment to hospitalization or illness
2. Promoting patient's comfort and hygiene
3. Contributing to medical treatment of patient
4. Arranging management details
5. Personal characteristics

On the basis of these lists of critical behaviors, a number of evaluation tools were developed including the Graphic Rating Form, behavioral checklists, a forced choice profile, and an observational record form.

Evaluating the Performance of Staff Nurses

Rosen and Abraham studied the Graphic Rating Form developed by Gorham *et al.* and then developed an evaluation procedure for assessing the performance of staff nurses.† Two evaluation methods were compared: one involved controlled manipulation of the variables and the systematic study of the outcomes; in the other, observations of critical incidents of on-the-job performance were collected. A form similar to the Graphic Rating Form was developed. The Nursing Performance Description Form (NPDF) was used to collect data about the performance of staff nurses. Criterion data were used in correlating performance ratings. The authors concluded that systematic evaluation using critical incidents could lead to important outcomes for hospital nursing programs, including improved communication, increased facilitation in making decisions, identification of developmental needs at various levels, recognition of merit, and identification of the roles of supervisory and staff personnel as well as other professional groups including medical residents.

* Gorham, Lichtenstein, and Marchese, *op. cit.*, p. 9.
† Albert Rosen and Gertrude E. Abraham. "Evaluation of a Procedure for Assessing the Performance of Staff Nurses," *Nursing Research*, 12:78-82, (Feb.) 1963.

A Global Evaluation Form was developed including a five-point scale for evaluating performance in the following areas:

1. Improving patients' adjustment to hospitalization or illness
2. Promoting patients' comfort and hygiene
3. Contributing to the medical treatment of patients
4. Arranging administrative details
5. Personal characteristics
6. Over-all effectiveness.*

Ratings on the NPDF and the Global Evaluation Form were compared. The most effective use of the two forms was achieved when a nurse, who was thoroughly familiar with the procedures, was available to assist and encourage head nurses to be objective in their ratings of staff personnel.

Reducing Medication Errors

The studies described above involved evaluation of over-all performance. The critical incident technique has also been used to identify behaviors in small units of work. Safren and Chapanis did a study of hospital medication errors. Information was collected from staff and patients in an 1100-bed hospital during a period of seven months.† A total of 178 critical incidents involving medication errors or near errors were reported. Some of the critical behaviors that Safren and Chapanis identified were:

1. Procedure for identifying the patient
2. Checking the medicine ticket against the patient's wristband
3. Checking physician's orders against nursing care cards and medicine tickets to detect discrepancies
4. Marking nursing care cards to indicate medicines to be poured when nurse leaves to pour them
5. Checking back and signing off when medications have been poured by others

In this study, critical incidents were analyzed to determine exactly what a nurse must do in administering medication.

Defining the Behavior of Mental Patients

Schmid did a study to provide a lay definition of mental illness.‡ He collected 854 critical incidents on the behavior of patients in mental hospitals using a "Patient Observational Record Form." Graduate nurses, student nurses, and nursing assistants were asked to describe incidents

---

* Rosen and Abraham, loc. cit.

† Miriam Safren and Alphonse Chapanis. "A Critical Study of Hospital Medication Errors," Hospitals, 34:32+, (May 1) 1960, and 34:53+, (May 16) 1960.

‡ John C. Flanagan and Fred W. Schmid. "The Critical Incident Approach to the Study of Psychopathology," J. Clin. Psychology, 15:136-39, 1959.

of observed behavior of mental patients in closed wards which suggested an improvement in the behavior of the patient; or, conversely, something observed which suggested need for further hospital help. The behaviors were classified into 108 categories; from these 14 major areas were identified in three groups: (1) aggressive vs. considerate behavior, (2) immature vs. mature behavior, and (3) irrational vs. rational behavior.

In a second study, Schmid had graduate nurses, student nurses, and nursing assistants record daily observations of critical incidents using a "Critical Behavior Record on Mental Patients." A total of 2972 critical behaviors were noted on patients who were primarily in privileged wards.*

These studies indicated that the critical incident technique could be used successfully in identifying behaviors of mental patients and in studies of psychopathology.

Behavioral Criteria for Effectiveness in Professional Nursing

Bailey collected 419 critical incidents from nursing supervisors, patients, and doctors on the behavior of professional staff nurses. Seven major behavior criteria of nursing effectiveness for professional, graduate, and staff were identified:

    I. Demonstrating manipulative skill and technical competence
    II. Demonstrating effective organization of work habits
    III. Performing effectively in an emergency or stress situation
    IV. Providing the patient with emotional support
    V. Demonstrating effective interpersonal relations with co-workers and visitors
    VI. Maintaining personal appearance and voice control
    VII. Demonstrating professionally ethical behavior†

In the statistical analysis of the incidents it was interesting to note that supervisory nurses most often contributed incidents relating to technical skill; doctors reported on incidents relating to performance in emergencies; whereas patients were most concerned with incidents involving emotional support.

This study indicated a very effective use of critical incidents in identifying criteria for performance in nursing.

Other applications of the critical incident technique to problems in nursing are cited at appropriate points later in the book.

At the present time the American Institutes for Research is engaged in several studies using critical incidents in nursing and related areas: (1) staff behaviors and mental retardate rehabilitation are being studied under a grant from the Department of Health, Education, and Welfare;

* Fred W. Schmid. "A Multidimensional Analysis of the Behavior of Hospitalized Mental Patients," unpublished doctoral dissertation, University of Pittsburgh, 1958.
† June Teig Bailey. "The Critical Incident Technique in Identifying Behavioral Criteria of Professional Nursing Effectiveness," *Nursing Research*, 5:52-64, (Oct.) 1956.

(2) a study of the use of critical incidents in teaching comprehensive medicine involving an evaluation of curricula in clinical medicine is being conducted for the American Association of Medical Colleges; and (3) a study of the identification of critical requirements for surgeons to be used to define competence in orthopedic surgery is being sponsored by the University of Illinois.* (See Appendix I.)

The critical incident technique is a versatile approach to the identification of behavior and critical requirements. Although further research will undoubtedly help to improve the procedures, at this point it has been established that critical incidents do provide verifiable, predictive information about performance in contrast to the random information usually collected from people in various fields who tend to talk about performance in terms of personal judgment and opinion rather than on the basis of direct observation of critical incidents of behavior.

STEP-BY-STEP PROCEDURES
IN USING THE
CRITICAL INCIDENT TECHNIQUE†

The critical incident technique is a method for collecting facts. What is an incident? *An incident is any observable bit of human behavior sufficiently complete in itself to permit inferences to be made about the person performing the act.*‡ Using this information, it may be assumed that all observable incidents about performance are facts. This is true. But, all facts are not incidents, and all incidents are not critical incidents. In order to be critical, an incident must make a significant difference in the outcome of the behavior; it must contribute either positively or negatively to the accomplishment of the aim of the activity.

If you should have occasion to participate in a critical incident research study, you will want to know:

1. How to define the aim or purpose of an activity. At the very beginning, before any data are collected, describe the purpose or aim of the activity. Data collectors and interviewees should have a common basis for understanding. A good definition can provide it. Statements of aim tend to vary from descriptions of operations to descriptions of equipment or people; often no aim or objective is specified. If data collection is to be successful, the aim or objective of the study must be clearly stated.

The statement of aim should be developed with care. The best ap-

* J. Michael Blum and Robert Fitzpatrick. *Critical Performance Requirements for Orthopedic Surgery*, Part I, "Method," American Institutes for Research, Pittsburgh, 1965.

† Information for this section of the book was derived mainly from an original article by John C. Flanagan on "The Critical Incident Technique," *Psychological Bulletin,* **51**:327-58, 1954.

‡ Flanagan, *loc. cit.*

proach is to collect information by talking with people who have had experience in the activity. Find out what they consider to be important. For example, if a decision is made to collect data for the evaluation of the performance of nursing students, talk with nursing educators and head nurses to determine what aspects of student and graduate nurse behavior they have observed and what they feel is important.

An exploratory interview could be conducted using an introductory statement such as:

> We are conducting a study to evaluate the performance of nursing students. We feel that you as an instructor (or head nurse) would be especially qualified to tell us about the behaviors you have observed which you feel are important.

Using the information provided in responses to this kind of question, the aim of a study to evaluate the behavior of nursing students might be as follows:

> The aim of this study is to collect critical incidents of the behavior of students who are giving nursing care to patients in the intensive care unit. This information will be used to evaluate performance and to develop an evaluation procedure.

2. How to develop plans and specifications. Once the aim of the study has been stated, make plans for collecting the data. Develop specifications regarding the kinds of information to be included.

a. *What situations are to be observed?* If behavior and performance of students in the intensive care unit are to be studied, indicate what aspects of performance in this unit are to be observed and recorded. If performance on more than one unit will be included, this should be specified. Instructors should be asked to think of the last time they observed a nursing student do something that was particularly effective. Ask them to describe what led up to the situation and exactly what happened. Then ask them to state why they felt the behavior was particularly effective. Ask for an example of ineffective behavior as well. In some instances, printed forms can be used, and instructors can record behaviors from actual observations during a one- or two-week period. Incidents should be recorded as soon as possible after they are observed.

b. *What is relevant?* It is sometimes difficult for an observer to decide whether or not a behavior has any relevance to the aim. For example, if an observer noted that a student prepared an excellent paper on teaching self-care to a diabetic patient, this would *not* be directly relevant to behavior on the intensive care unit. The observer would record an effective incident for the preparation of a paper on diabetic self-care. However, the incident would have no relevance to the student's performance on the intensive care unit. On the other hand, if the student had been observed adjusting an airway when she noted a postoperative patient was having difficulty in breathing, this *would* have direct relevance to behavior in the intensive care unit.

c. *What was the extent of the effect of the behavior?* Often when people observe behavior, they have difficulty deciding *how important the behavior was* and to what extent it affected the success or failure of the outcome. Critical incidents are those that make a significant difference in the positive or negative outcome of an activity. All behaviors are not critical. Adequacy of the behavior is also important. The incident must be *sufficiently* important to make a difference in the outcome.* For example: In taking a patient's temperature, if the student shakes down the thermometer and inserts it under the patient's tongue but does nothing more, this is *insufficient*. No decision can be made about the effect of this behavior until the nurse follows through and removes the thermometer from the patient's mouth after a time lapse of three minutes. She should *read* the temperature from the thermometer and record it on the patient's record. If she follows through and records the temperature accurately, she has completed the task in a satisfactory manner. However, if she makes an error in recording the temperature and writes down 102.2° instead of 99.2° this is the kind of an error that *could make a significant difference* in the treatment of the patient.

If a senior student noted infiltration into the tissue during an infusion and stopped the flow of the solution, it would be a behavior that was sufficiently effective to relieve a great deal of pain and prevent damage to body tissue.

d. *How to select observers.* Observers are very important in a critical incident study. They should be well qualified and trained to make observations in accordance with certain specifications. The best observers are usually people who supervise or direct the work being studied. Instructors and head nurses make the best observers if the information being collected concerns the behavior of nursing students. If it is not possible to use instructors or head nurses, other people can be trained to become good observers, provided they thoroughly understand what they are to do, how they are to go about it, and how to record what they observe.

3. How to collect the data. After plans and specifications have been developed and observers have been selected and taught how to collect critical incidents, the real work can begin. Emphasize the fact that incidents should be recorded as soon as possible after they have been observed. Don't let an incident grow cold. Time blurs or obliterates details and memory can distort the facts.

---

* Hobert W. Burns. "The Critical Incident Technique as an Instrument of Educational Research: A Philosophical Analysis," unpublished doctoral dissertation, Stanford University, 1957. Doctoral Dissertation Series Publication No. 25:345, p. 277 (University of Michigan Microfilming Service).

In some preliminary studies it may be necessary to collect incidents based on memory; if so, observers should be asked to record only recent incidents, and a time limit should be set to write incidents that occurred no more than a week or two weeks before the record is written.

If a form is devised and observers are asked to record incidents *as they occur,* or as soon thereafter as possible, more accurate data can be collected. The form should ask the following questions: Did you observe a nurse doing something effective (or ineffective) today? What led up to the situation? Exactly what happened? Why was the behavior considered effective (or ineffective)?

a. *How many incidents are needed to do a critical incident study?* This can vary depending on the nature of the project. In studies involving supervision of other personnel it was found that between 2000 and 4000 incidents were needed. Where production work was involved, fewer incidents were needed. The adequacy of the sample can be determined on the basis of a preliminary classification of the incidents.

b. *How are the data classified?* Collect several hundred incidents and appoint someone on the research staff to begin sorting the incidents into related groups. This is done by separating them into stacks on the basis of the behaviors involved. Put all the incidents that describe one kind of behavior together; those describing other types of behavior should be placed in separate piles.

Classification is achieved on the basis of inductive reasoning. For example, if the critical incidents are going to be used for evaluation purposes, the frame of reference should be on-the-job effectiveness and the categories should refer to behaviors relating to effectiveness and criteria for success in nursing.

c. *How to formulate the categories.* This step requires a good deal of insight and experience. There are no simple rules. Although there tends to be a great deal of subjectivity in this process, it is possible to overcome it to a degree. The thing to do is to submit the list of categories to other qualified persons for their review. This does not guarantee the success of a set of objective categories, but at least it introduces the possibility for disagreement or an impartial suggestion if there are apparent oversights. Of course, even experts tend to differ about degrees of importance in various behaviors; still it has been shown there can be considerable inter-rater reliability when a number of people rate the behaviors of a given group.* The test of the justification for formulating the categories is: Does the categorization scheme really serve its purpose?† Does it separate behaviors into the categories that are *important?*

After the initial separation of a sample of the incidents, label the groups

* Joy P. Guilford *et al.* "Ratings Should Be Scrutinized." *Educational and Psychological Measurement,* 22:439-47, 1962.
† Burns, *op. cit.,* p. 277.

in a tentative way and define the kinds of behavior to be included in each. For example, in a study where an evaluation tool for nursing behavior is to be developed, some of the tentative categories might be (1) developing plans for nursing care, (2) checking orders, (3) interpersonal relationships. Trial separations of the incidents should be made using these tentative categories. At some point it may appear that there are enough subgroups within a major area to warrant a separation. For example, under the main heading "Checking Orders" it may develop that there are numerous incidents about checking medication cards. If so, a subgroup should be identified to include incidents of this type.

After the sample sorting using the tentative behavior categories, some additional incidents should be classified. If it becomes necessary to broaden the coverage of a category to include a few more relevant behaviors, don't hesitate to do it. On the other hand, there may be two kinds of behavior involved in one category that appear to be of equal importance. If so, separate these into two distinct categories. This refinement and modification of the category headings may go through several stages. When you discover that adding another 100 or 200 incidents yields only one or two rather minor kinds of variation, it is fairly safe to decide that enough incidents have been collected to reflect a representative sample of the behaviors involved in a given activity.

4. How to analyze the data. If the first three steps of the study go well, and you collect a representative sample of incidents, it should be possible to analyze the data without too much difficulty. The main purpose of the analysis is to make the data more useful, to develop a statement of the critical requirements of the activity being studied, and to summarize the information so that it can serve a practical purpose.

Data analysis involves three important steps:

Establishing the frame of reference
Inductively developing the categories of behaviors for use in classifying
    the incidents
Identifying and describing the critical requirements of the activity

a. *How to establish the frame of reference.* As indicated earlier, critical incidents can be used for a variety of purposes including establishing criteria, measuring typical performance, and developing measures of proficiency. No single frame of reference can be identified as the absolute *right* one, but it is possible to determine the *appropriate* one for a particular study. The decision has to be made on the basis of the purposes for which the information will be used. This assumes that the aim of the activity has been specifically stated and defined in a clear-cut statement.

b. *How to formulate the categories.* Flanagan states:

The induction of categories from the basic data in the form of incidents is a task requiring insight, experience, and judgment. Unfortunately, this procedure is, in the present state of psychological knowledge, more subjective than objective.*

The skill and sophistication of the researcher play an important part in this phase of a critical incident study.

One important test of the appropriateness of the categories that are developed is to submit them to several experts in the activity to make certain that the scheme is doing what it set out to do, that is, to describe all aspects of the behaviors in the activity.

An important consideration in the inductive development of categories for classifying incidents is to ask the question: Do the critical requirements describe the behaviors represented by the sample of incidents collected, and could they also be used to predict future behaviors in this activity?†

If the categories described can be used to predict future behavior, then you've done it! The categorization scheme worked. If, on the other hand, the behavioral statements are not predictive of future behavior in this same activity, you will need to retrace your steps and re-examine the categories to determine whether greater specificity is needed in the statements about the behaviors, or whether the aim of the study was too broadly stated.

Decisions about the amount of detail to include or exclude should be made on the basis of the ultimate use of the information. If a set of critical requirements for an activity is to be developed, a great deal of specificity is desirable, and subcategories should be identified and described. On the other hand, if the information is to be used in a broad, general way, only the broader aspects of the behavior need to be described.

Flanagan suggests several points to be remembered in describing behavior or critical requirements in the classification scheme.‡

1. The headings or captions should be logically organized.
2. The titles of the headings should be clear enough that no lengthy explanations of their meanings are needed.
3. The language used in the headings should be parallel in structure and content.
4. The headings should represent relatively the same levels of importance.
5. The headings should be comprehensive enough to cover all the incidents that would fall into each category.

   c. *How to describe critical requirements.* The statements of behavior should be as specific and descriptive as possible. The information derived

---

* Flanagan, *op. cit.*, p. 344.
† Burns, *op. cit.*, p. 277.
‡ Flanagan, *op. cit.*, p. 344.

from the list of categories should be useful in describing the critical requirements of an activity, because each category contains a list of the
behaviors that have been found to be important to the aim of the activity.
These should be the critical behaviors that one would seek in a situation
involving selection of a person for training in a particular activity, or in
making a decision regarding advanced education or job training, depending
on the purpose for which the critical behaviors are described.

For example, Barham collected critical incidents for the purpose of determining behaviors important to effective instruction in nursing. The behaviors she developed included the following:*

1. Accepting students as individuals
2. Admitting limitations honestly
3. Avoiding humiliating student in front of others
4. Being available when appropriate
5. Counseling without humiliating
6. Demonstrating confidence in the student
7. Demonstrating flexibility so that learning can take place
8. Demonstrating understanding in working with student
9. Empathizing with student
10. Establishing rapport with student
11. Exhibiting appropriate preparation
12. Explaining for understanding
13. Giving student feeling of importance
14. Going into problem situation with student
15. Producing a defensive response
16. Recognizing individual needs
17. Setting an example
18. Showing restraint so that own anxiety does not influence situation
19. Stimulating and involving students

5. How to interpret and report the findings. The final step in using
critical incidents is the interpretation and reporting of the findings. In many
studies, the first four steps may be carried out efficiently; however, it may
be difficult to report the findings accurately. Be honest and a bit humble.
State the limitations of the sample used—if there are certain limitations.
Avoid broad generalizations.

For example, effective teaching in a school of nursing may require a
somewhat different set of critical requirements than effective teaching in a
school of drama; and critical behaviors for competent nursing will differ
markedly from the critical behaviors for success as a microbiologist. Therefore, generalizing a set of critical behaviors from one activity to another

---

* Virginia Z. Barham. "Identifying Effective Behavior of the Nursing Instructor
through Critical Incidents," *Nursing Research*, 14:67, (Winter) 1965.

activity may fall far short of the mark if the conditions of the two activities are not comparable.

The critical requirements determined in any one study cannot be assumed to cover every phase of a group of activities; they are, in fact, rather specific to the particular activity described. However, it is possible to generalize to the extent that the critical requirements identified for effective teaching in a sample of representative schools of nursing could be generalized to predict behaviors appropriate for success in effective instruction in comparable schools of nursing.

The skill, good judgment, and insight of the researcher, as well as a recognition of the limitations involved, play an important part in the interpretation of the findings in a study. It is the obligation of the researcher to report his findings as accurately as possible based on his judgment of the implications of his research for practical purposes.

These are the steps involved in using the critical incident technique for research purposes. In the chapters that follow the technique will be applied to some of the key problems in nursing education:

1. The identification of the objectives in a school of nursing
2. Curriculum development and the organization of learning experiences
3. Evaluating the performance of students and practitioners
4. Relating performance to professional standards

Bibliography

American Institutes for Research. A *Report of Three Years of Experience,* American Institutes for Research, Pittsburgh, 1950.

Bailey, June T. "The Critical Incident Technique in Identifying Behavioral Criteria of Professional Nursing Effectiveness," *Nursing Research,* 5:52-64, (Oct.) 1956.

Barham, Virginia Z. "Identifying Effective Behavior of the Nursing Instructor through Critical Incidents," *Nursing Research,* 14:66-77, (Winter) 1965.

Blum, J. Michael, and Fitzpatrick, Robert. *Critical Performance Requirements for Orthopedic Surgery, Part I,* "*Method,*" American Institutes for Research, Pittsburgh, 1965.

Burns, Hobert W. "The Critical Incident Technique as an Instrument of Educational Research: A Philosophical Analysis," unpublished doctoral dissertation, Stanford University, 1957. (Available on microfilm from the University of Michigan in Doctoral Dissertation Series Publication No. 25:345.)

Flanagan, John C. "The Critical Incident Technique," *The Psychological Bulletin,* 51:327-58, 1954.

Flanagan, John C. "The Aviation Psychology Program in the Army Air Forces," *Army Air Forces Aviation Psychology Program Research Report No. 1,* U.S. Government Printing Office, Washington, D.C., 1947.

Flanagan, John C., and Schmid, F. W. "The Critical Incident Approach to the Study of Psychopathology," *J. Clin. Psychology,* 15:136-39, 1959.

Flanagan, John C. et al. *Critical Requirements for Research Personnel,* American Institutes for Research, Pittsburgh, 1949.

Gorham, William A., and Lichtenstein, Stanley. *Specific Nursing Behaviors Related to Patient Care and Improvement*, American Institutes for Research, Washington, D.C., 1959 (AIR-B24-59).

Gorham, William A., Lichtenstein, Stanley, and Marchese, Angeline C. *Specific Nursing Behaviors Related to Patient Care and Improvement: Measuring Nursing Performance*, American Institutes for Research, Pittsburgh, and Washington, D.C., 1959 (AIR-B-24-59-FR-204).

Guilford, Joy P. *et al.* "Ratings Should Be Scrutinized," *Educational and Psychological Measurement*, **22**:439-47, 1962.

Preston, Harley O. *The Development of a Procedure for Evaluating Officers in the United States Air Force*, American Institutes for Research, Pittsburgh, 1948. (Report includes a checklist of critical requirements.)

Pumroy, Shirley S., and Suttell, Barbara J. *The Private Duty Nurse: Her Role in the Hospital Environment of Washington, D.C.*, American Institutes for Research, Washington, D.C., 1956 (AIR-B3-56-FR-136).

Rosen, Albert, and Abraham, Gertrude E. "Evaluation of a Procedure for Assessing the Performance of Staff Nurses," *Nursing Research*, **12**:78-82, (Feb.) 1963.

Safren, Miriam, and Chapanis, Alphonse. "A Critical Study of Hospital Medication Errors," *Hospitals*, **34**:32+, (May 1) 1960 and **34**:53+, (May 16) 1960.

Schmid, Fred W. "A Multidimensional Analysis of the Behavior of Hospitalized Mental Patients," unpublished doctoral dissertation, University of Pittsburgh, 1958.

Weislogel, Mary H. *Evaluating the Performance of Research Personnel: A Manual for Supervisors*, American Institutes for Research, Pittsburgh, 1951 (AIR-A33-51-PR-13).

Selected References

(Note: These references include studies using the critical incident technique in a variety of situations: teaching, evaluation, motivation, counseling, psychotherapy, selection, and in the identification of critical requirements.)

Blair, J. R. "Classroom Effectiveness of Teaching as Perceived by High School Students," unpublished doctoral dissertation, University of Mississippi, 1962.

Cooper, Bernice. "Critical Requirements for Principalship Based on Critical Incidents of Instructors, Supervisors, and Visiting Teachers," unpublished doctoral dissertation, University of Georgia, 1955.

Domas, Sidney J. *Report of an Exploratory Study of Teacher Competence*, New England School Development Council, Cambridge, Mass., 1950.

Eilbert, Leo R. "A Study of Emotional Immaturity Utilizing the Critical Incident Technique," University of Pittsburgh Bulletin, **49**:199-204, 1953.

Fitzpatrick, Robert. *A Pilot Study of Factors Which Influence the Cancer Patient's Choice of Medical Treatment*, American Institutes for Research, Pittsburgh, 1955. (AIR-B10-55-FR-107).

Flanagan, John C. "Defining the Requirements of the Executive's Job," *Personnel*, **28**:28-35, 1951.

Flanagan, John C. "Principles and Procedures in Evaluating Performance," *Personnel*, **28**:373-86, 1952.

Goldin, M. "Behaviors Related to Effective Teaching," unpublished doctoral dissertation, University of Wisconsin, 1957.

Greenberg, M. S. "Patient Reported Disturbances in the Hospital Treatment of Cancer Patients as Elicited by the Critical Incident Technique," unpublished master's thesis, University of Houston, 1961.

Gropper, George L. *The Critical Requirements of Conference Behavior*, Maynard Foundation, Pittsburgh, 1956.

Hahn, Clifford P. "The Identification and Description of Some Critical Aircrew Job Requirements," USAF School of Aviation Medicine Report No. 2, Project No. RDB 2102-174, 1954 (AIR-A24-54-IR-24).

Harrington, R. J. "Critical Requirements of Ward Attendants," unpublished master's thesis, University of New Hampshire, 1957.

Hedlund, P. A. "Cooperative Study to Predict Effectiveness in Secondary School Teaching," *J. Teacher Education*, 4:230-34, 1953.

Herzberg, F., Inkley, S., and Adams, W. R. "Some Effects on the Clinical Faculty of a Critical Incident Study of the Performance of Students," *J. Med. Education*, 35:666-74, 1960.

Herzberg, F., Mausner, B., and Snyderman, B. *The Motivation to Work*, John Wiley & Sons, Inc., New York, 1959.

Jensen, A. C. "Determining Critical Requirements for Teachers," *J. Exper. Education*, 20:79-86, 1951.

Lewis, Garland K. "The Use of a Modified Critical Incident Technique in the Identification of Functions of Psychiatric Aide in a Private Psychiatric Hospital," unpublished master's thesis, University of Washington, 1958.

Mayhew, L. B. "The Critical Incident Technique in Educational Evaluation," *J. Educational Research*, 49:591-98, 1956.

Nelson, K. G., Bicknell, J. E., and Hedlund, P. A. *Development and Refinement of Measures of Teaching Effectiveness*, State Education Department, University of New York, 1956.

O'Donnell, R. J. "The Development and Evaluation of a Test for Predicting Dental Student Performance," *University of Pittsburgh Bulletin*, 49:240-45, 1953.

Schmid, D. B., and Cohen, D. "The Selection of Psychiatric Aides: I. Critical Requirements of the Job," *Am. J. Psychiat.* 112:451-56, 1955.

Schwarz, P. A. *Critical Requirements for Pharmaceutical Representatives*, American Institutes for Research, Pittsburgh, 1958 (AIR-B-52-58-FR).

Stewart, L. H. "Critical Training Requirements for Teaching Success," *J. Educational Research*, 49:651-61, 1956.

Wager, C. E., and Sharon, M. I. "Defining Job Requirements in Terms of Behavior," *Personnel Admin.*, 14:18-25, 1951.

Wagner, R. F. "A Study of the Critical Requirements for Dentists," *University of Pittsburgh Bulletin*, 46:331-39, 1950.

Weissman, I., and Baker, Mary R. *Education for Social Workers in the Public Social Services*, Council on Social Work Education, New York, 1959.

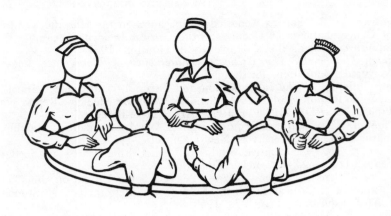

Critical Incident

At a meeting of the curriculum committee there was a review of course objectives for purposes of revising them to provide the basis for developing course content and selecting related learning experiences. It was suggested that the committee include a learning experience covering the outpatient department. However, this particular school of nursing did not have an outpatient department as part of its facility.

Miss Dunn, the Medical-Surgical Coordinator, suggested the possibility of using the expanded outpatient facilities of a nearby medical center hospital and offered to help make arrangements to do this. She also suggested that the Public Health Coordinator be consulted in developing the course objectives and content consistent with the outpatient experience.

This was an effective critical incident for Miss Dunn. She first identified a facility that would serve the needs of the school and was alert to recognize that with modern trends in medical and nursing care plans the student should be knowledgeable about and gain experience in various types of clinics. She demonstrated knowledge of community health facilities and volunteered to assist in exploring the possibility for using them. In this way she contributed to the possible enrichment of the nursing education program for students in that school.

Chapter 3
The Critical Requirements
Approach to
Establishing Objectives in a
School of Nursing

The critical requirements approach has potential for solutions to problems in the field of nursing education. It is not a panacea for all our problems, but a systematic data-collection method of this type is one way to gather relevant facts and analyze them objectively.

Flanagan proposed that any list of educational objectives should be—

> . . . simply stated in terms which can readily be comprehended and agreed to by typical parents and citizens . . . that a preliminary set of critical requirements be developed on the basis of aptitude, ability, attitude, or other requirement[s].*

He suggested the advisability of seeking the cooperative efforts of people who are qualified to assist in establishing objectives, such as appropriate representatives from the community, from industry, and from other interested agencies.

Objectives in a school of nursing are developed by a committee whose judgment and knowledge of the school and its philosophy and purposes provide the basis for decisions regarding the desired outcomes of the educational program. In addition to the capability of the committee on objectives, Flanagan† suggests the desirability of going beyond the point of collecting information just from those closest to the problem. Facts should be collected from other people engaged directly and indirectly in the activity—teachers, students, members of the community served by the school, representatives of industry served by the graduates of the school, and other interested citizens. People from these groups can serve as consultants to the committee on objectives.

* John C. Flanagan. "The Critical-Requirements Approach to Educational Objectives," *School and Society*, 71:321-24, 1950, p. 321.
† Flanagan, *loc. cit.*

The method proposed for gathering information from these sources is to use questionnaires similar to those described in Chapter 2. Interviews would be held individually or in groups with people whose interests are served by the school and who, as such, would be asked to express their views of the objectives the school should achieve. Because critical incidents are reports of observed facts, the questions asked during the interviews would be behaviorally centered around the nurse who represents the product or outcome of the educational environment in a school of nursing.

A study of this type would be designed to elicit from consultants in community health, industrial nursing, and related agencies, as well as users of nursing service, specific incidents of effective and ineffective behavior they had observed on the part of nurses giving patient care in hospitals, rehabilitation centers, or health clinics.

Several stipulations should be made about the sample from whom these incidents would be collected:

1. The incidents reported would be on the basis of actual behavior observed.
2. The observers would be those who have a knowledge of the aims and goals of the individual with respect to the activity observed.
3. The judgments to be made by the observers in applying the criteria for determining especially effective or ineffective behavior would be clearly defined.
4. The observers would be persons qualified to make judgments regarding successful and unsuccessful behavior in the activity observed.
5. The conditions of reporting would need to be such as to ensure a reasonable degree of accuracy.

These are the conditions set forth by Flanagan in proposing a study to collect information to help in the formulation of general educational objectives.* These conditions could be used in a study to formulate objectives for a school of nursing. Plans for such a study, of course, would require participation by representatives of the school of nursing working in close cooperation with researchers knowledgeable in nursing. The formulation of questionnaires for the data-gathering phase of the study would require the cooperative efforts of both. The approach to analysis of the incidents would be somewhat similar to that described in Chapter 2. Several other questions should be answered before such a study could be undertaken.

WHY DEFINE OBJECTIVES?

Before objectives for a school of nursing can be defined, it is necessary to decide what we mean by objectives and what purpose they serve. Teachers

* Flanagan, *op. cit.*, p. 322.

have taught for years without statements of educational goals, and some have been quite successful. Why is it important to define objectives?

First, let us consider what we hope to achieve as a result of an educational program. If teachers were asked to summarize educational achievement in a single word, that word might well be *learning*. Teachers hope for some demonstration of learning. In a school of nursing we hope students will learn to become competent nurses.

Educators, psychologists, and behavioral scientists have spent a great deal of time trying to define *learning*. To date the most comprehensive and accepted definitions imply that *learning results when specific kinds of changes take place in the behavior of the student*. For example, at one point a child cannot read; after some instruction he may identify certain simple words. This shows he now can read words he could not read before instruction. He has *learned to read simple words*. The same is true when a child is first given a series or set of numbers. He may be able to identify each as an isolated number, but he may know nothing about adding or subtracting them. After some instruction he may be able to add and subtract simple numbers. Again, some learning has taken place—there is a demonstrated change in the student's behavior from not knowing what to do to being able to work with numbers and apply elementary principles of arithmetic.

In nursing, we have a similar situation. One day a student knows what a thermometer is, but she has never used one. After a demonstration of correct procedures, she may be able to read the thermometer and take temperatures in several ways. She has learned to take temperatures using thermometers.

But, the word *learning* has tremendously broad, encompassing, and sometimes ambiguous implications. It can cover a wide range of behaviors from the simple addition or subtraction of two-digit numbers to the use of advanced mathematical principles required to solve complex problems in physics; or from learning to give back rubs to solving or helping patients to solve covert problems in meeting emotional needs. For this reason, objectives of a nursing education program cannot be defined simply by stating that we expect a demonstration of learning. More complete and comprehensive objectives are required—statements that describe the types of changes we expect in the student, the kinds of concepts and principles she should understand and be able to use, and the nature of the patient care she should be able to give when she graduates.

These objectives must be established at several levels:

1. Broad, general statements are needed to develop programs of instruction, to describe the types of courses and the subject areas to be covered, and to establish the kinds of general goals toward which programs of education should aim.
2. Behavioral objectives should be established at the second level. Here

the intent is to help analyze the broad, general goals into more specific aims to be used in the development of curriculums. At this level the purpose is to specify the goals of instruction in terms of courses, units, or general segments, and the sequencing of these to achieve the general objectives of the program.

3. At the third level, objectives are needed for the development of instructional materials that will help to achieve specific unit, lesson, or course objectives.

These are the three levels on which objectives should be established if educational goals are to be achieved. When defined in behavioral terms, goals at the second and third levels should provide guidance to teachers in teaching and to students in learning; thus directed, it should be possible for both to achieve the general objectives of the educational program.

The basic reason for defining objectives is to provide guidance for teacher and student activities in the educational process.

WHAT ARE THE PURPOSES
OF EDUCATIONAL OBJECTIVES?

Objectives serve to integrate activities of each of the various levels of education so that it is possible to achieve the ultimate aim or goal of the program. The objectives of a lesson or a unit help to achieve the objectives of sections of the curriculum which, in turn, when integrated with the curriculums at succeeding levels, help to achieve the general goal of the school.

Tyler identifies three important purposes of educational objectives:*

1. *Objectives should serve as a guide to teacher behavior.* Many teachers present curriculum content effectively and their students demonstrate evidence of learning by passing qualifying exams. These teachers may feel no need for statements of objectives; they may have goals in mind but have never developed them in written form. For most teachers, however, statements of objectives can be quite important for guidance in teaching.

When contractors build a high-rise apartment building, their first requirement is an architectural design. Given the design, they need plans and specifications describing in detail each aspect of the design and how it can be achieved. In nursing education, the over-all design is the competent nurse. To achieve this goal, educators need detailed plans and specifications in the form of objectives for the curriculums and the courses they teach. Objectives can serve to guide nurse educators in teaching students to become competent nurses.

2. *Objectives can assist in orienting and guiding the student.* If students

---

* Ralph W. Tyler, "Some Persistent Questions on the Defining of Objectives," in C. M. Lindvall (ed.). *Defining Educational Objectives*, University of Pittsburgh Press, 1964, pp. 77-83.

are to achieve their goals, they, too, need to know what they are expected to achieve as a result of taking specific courses. Without objectives it is difficult for them to realize what they are to do with the information they are learning. For example, in a school of nursing, students frequently feel it is sufficient to read and review textbook materials until they can pass a test. In some cases this may satisfy the student because she does pass a final examination and gets a satisfactory grade in a course. If no other objective is stated, the student can only assume that the main objective is to pass the course. But there is more to nursing education than merely passing courses.

When the student is presented with statements of objectives for a course, she becomes aware of the kinds of changes in her behavior she should be able to demonstrate when she completes that course. In an introductory unit on medical-surgical nursing the student should learn fundamental skills; the statement of objectives should contain information to this effect supported by an explanation of the specific skills the student should be expected to demonstrate when she completes the course. Merely being able to answer questions on a paper-and-pencil test or in an oral examination about medical-surgical nursing would not be regarded as sufficient. The student should be able to demonstrate in actual practice that she can apply skills required to give adequate, safe patient-centered care in an intensive care unit.

Mager and McCann found that students who had statements of objectives at the outset of a course tended to complete the requirements and achieve the objectives in a shorter time than those who merely attended classes throughout the term without knowing what they were expected to do as a result of taking the course.*

Tyler contends that by presenting students with statements of objectives we are not attempting to give them all the answers—we are endeavoring to establish goals the student can understand and use to guide and organize her own learning activities.†

3. *Objectives can help instructors to assess student progress.* When objectives are clear-cut, teachers can make estimates of progress toward those goals. Teaching is a complex process; it is not possible to develop simple, "pat" sets of rules or formulas on how to teach—each group of students and each teaching situation requires special treatment. However, teachers can use statements of objectives to develop plans for teaching and to determine how well the students are learning the materials in a given program. It is possible to judge whether the objectives of the program are being met, how far the students have progressed, and how far they must go to reach the goal.

* Robert F. Mager and Joseph McCann. *Learner Controlled Instruction,* Varian Associates, Palo Alto, 1961.
† Tyler, *op. cit.,* p. 83.

WHO SHOULD ESTABLISH
OBJECTIVES?

Clarification of the objectives of an educational program in a school of nursing requires the work of people at all levels. Standardizing agencies, prominent educators, psychologists, school administrators, subject-matter teachers, and qualified citizens in a community all have a role to play in the process. At the national level, broad, general statements of the objectives of the nursing profession are formulated by representative agencies. However, there is great need for further clarification and definition in terms of school objectives. What is expected in the way of outcomes? What means and methods can be used to achieve the goals? What kinds of behavioral changes will be accepted as evidence that goals have been reached?

Gagné summarized educational goals into three major areas:

Education has the purpose of making it possible for the individual to participate in and to share with other people in a variety of aesthetic experiences.

A second major goal is the development of responsible citizenship.

The development of individual talents to the end of achieving satisfaction in a life work or vocation is a third goal.*

Gagné indicates, however, that these are not sufficient. He feels we should analyze and break them down into smaller units or components and stipulate steps leading toward specific goals. How will the information and knowledge the student acquires in one course relate to later experiences in school, in a career, and in life?

Reducing broad, general objectives to small components shifts the responsibility from national levels to local groups familiar with the specific educational needs of particular schools of nursing. Faculty committees in various fields within individual schools should assume responsibility for refining broad objectives. In nursing it is the obligation of educators within the profession working cooperatively with representative groups from the community—

1. To establish objectives consistent with the general goals of nursing
2. To develop objectives appropriate for each type of educational program (vocational, associate degree, diploma, and collegiate)
3. To develop the curriculum and specify course content
4. To establish criteria for acceptable standards of performance required

* Robert M. Gagné. "Educational Objectives and Human Performance," chapter in *Learning and the Educational Process* by John Krumboltz. Rand McNally & Company, Chicago, 1965.

to meet the objectives of each type of program, together with lists of the behaviors expected

5. To adopt suitable techniques for assessing or evaluating both teacher and student progress in relation to established goals

Researchers in education, in psychology, and in nursing have conducted studies investigating activities in many professional fields. Their findings are available and can be used to develop procedures for identifying and achieving objectives in a school of nursing. But, the primary responsibility in any nursing education program rests with the members of the faculty and educational administrators of that school.

WHAT ARE SOME BASIC CONSIDERATIONS IN DEFINING OBJECTIVES?

Too many goals cause confusion; goals that are too broad leave doubt; and goals that are not specific are difficult to achieve. Dressel cites three needs that should guide committees in developing objectives:

. . . the needs of society, the needs of the individual, and authority.*

He cautions that a great many unrelated objectives may result. To help to overcome the problem he suggests that educators work to define objectives that will be—

. . . 1) reasonable in number; 2) consistent with one another; 3) of approximately the same level of generality or specificity; 4) distinctive . . . although not completely independent; and 5) descriptive of goals verifiably achievable by the means at hand.†

The committee on objectives should try to develop goals that are student-centered rather than teacher-centered. Nursing education goals should not be determined solely on the basis of how much material an instructor can present in a given period of time, but rather in terms of how much and what kinds of materials a student should be able to learn, as demonstrated by specific changes in behavior.

Tyler refers to five basic considerations important in the development of educational objectives:‡

1. *What are the needs of our culture?* It is important to teach the kinds of behavior, the ways of thinking, feeling, and acting that have value in our society and that will help a person to behave effectively in our culture. For example, in teaching nursing skills to students who plan to practice nursing

---

* Paul L. Dressel and associates. *Evaluation in Higher Education,* Houghton Mifflin Company, Boston, 1961, p. 12.

† Dressel, *loc. cit.*

‡ Tyler, *op. cit.,* pp. 79-81.

in remote South American villages, a very different set of values and skills would be required from those needed by a student who plans a career as a nurse in a large, modern American hospital. A survey of requirements should include not only the needs of the culture and society in general, but the specific health needs of the community as well. For example, the nursing needs in an industrial city would center around industrial health problems. Students who will practice nursing in these areas should have experiences planned in cooperation with an industrial health clinic.

2. *What is the student ready to learn?* What has the student learned up to this point? What background does she bring to the learning situation? What is she ready to learn next? There are wide individual differences among students. Many students learn at a pace nearly twice as fast as the average students in a class.* Some learn in the sense that they can recall the facts and repeat them, but they can do little beyond that. Others can make practical application of the principles and information they have learned. At the upper end of a class there may be some who have progressed far beyond the beginning level in a course of instruction; whereas at the lower end there will be some who lack the prerequisites needed to learn even the most elementary concepts.

Saupe states:

> . . . the determination of the readiness . . . of individual students and the planning of instruction . . . require . . . assessment of student characteristics . . . [and the] study of the effectiveness of the various educational experiences which have been planned in relation to the readiness characteristics observed.†

Learning experiences should build upon one another in a way that continued learning and reinforcement take place. The student should be given opportunities to apply what she has learned in initial or beginning courses to the work she must do at advanced levels in nursing education. This assumes, of course, that some learning of related materials has taken place earlier in the student's experience.

Tyler states:

> . . . a key problem in selecting objectives is that of determining the "entering behavior" of a student, just where [she] is in [her] educational development and what abilities [she] brings to the given class or learning situation.‡

For example, it would be somewhat unrealistic to expect the student to be able to administer drugs intelligently to a patient if she had not first been

---

* John C. Flanagan *et al. The American High School Student,* Houghton Mifflin Company, Boston, in press.
† Paul L. Dressel and associates, *op. cit.,* Chapter 3, "Learning and Evaluation Processes," by Joe L. Saupe, p. 57.
‡ Tyler, *op. cit.,* p. 80.

exposed to information in relation to the classification of drugs, their action, minimal and maximal dosage, and the technique of administration.

Instructors should use achievement tests and actual demonstrations to determine what the student has already learned in order to decide on the next steps in education. For example, it would be unrealistic to expect a student to try to learn how to instruct a patient in home and self-care if she had not learned something about effective communication. Or, it would be unreasonable to present the student with a problem in briefing a patient and preparing her for a radical mastectomy if the student had not studied some psychology and had not learned how to assist the patient in meeting emotional problems.

Learning new information is often contingent upon past learning experience. It is important to know what knowledge the student has in order to plan logically for next steps to be taken. Allowances must be made for the individual differences that exist not only in previous learning, but in capacity to learn new information. Every student will not have the same degree of readiness regardless of identical learning experiences. Within a single class there will be many variations in (1) the amount of information the student learns, (2) the degree of capability in relating new information and new concepts to previous learning, (3) the power of retention for future use, (4) the ability to recall appropriate information required to learn the new lesson, (5) the ability to generalize, and (6) the capability for "discovering" new concepts.

3. *What can we teach?* We should be aware of the limitations of present knowledge in certain fields. For example, it would be ideal if nursing instructors could teach students the reasons why there are subtle physical or emotional changes in patients who are being given new drugs. Early identification of allergic reactions would be very desirable. It would be well if we could tell the student why such reactions occur. At this point we only know that they *do* occur; unfortunately, we do not yet know *why*.

In another area, as a result of recent new knowledge, we can teach students the use of electronic devices such as the improved oxygen tents, the cardiac pacemaker-monitor, and other innovations in patient care. Devices have been developed to monitor the condition of 12 patients simultaneously through a console that electronically records patients' pulse rates, respiration rates, temperatures, and blood pressure readings. Telemetry has made it possible to introduce some important changes in patient monitoring based on innovations of the space age.* Another electronic advance monitors, measures, and controls the flow of intravenous infusions. This device helps prevent the possibility of fatal air embolisms; an automatic shut-off pinches the tube, preventing air flow into the patient's veins.

---

* Clair D. O'Malley. "Nursing in a Space-Age Hospital," *Am. J. Nursing*, **62**:54-58, (Dec.), 1962.

These are just a few of the changes, innovations, and scientific advances in equipment and methods for patient care that are available now and can be part of what we teach today; tomorrow the state of our knowledge will change. Educational objectives in nursing should be reviewed periodically and updated to include new findings. Changes in the field should be examined to determine what is new and to assess its value. Every effort should be made to incorporate the new information into educational programs if and when it is feasible. The best way to prepare nursing students with a working knowledge of up-to-date information in patient care, nursing education, and nursing research is through continuous re-evaluation and review of objectives at all levels.

4. *Is the objective relevant to the educational philosophy of the school?* Tyler states:

. . . the philosophy of a school outlines the concept of the "good person" we are trying to develop.*

Educational objectives in a school of nursing should be consistent with the concept of the *good nurse* the school hopes to develop. Committees on objectives should establish goals that are realistic for the students to attain and that represent the kinds of achievement which will enable students to become competent nurses.

5. *Is the objective consistent with current values?* There are many values to be realized in education and many levels on which learning can be achieved. On one hand there is the notion that every effort should be made to educate young people in basic occupational skills so that they can become productive citizens in our society. This implies providing only the bare essentials so that people will become self-supporting members of a community with a sense of respect for leadership. This is what Tyler describes as the "garden variety" of citizen.* These people must leave leadership and the exploration of new knowledge to a privileged few who cultivate their capabilities. To assume that the growing needs for nursing service can be filled by technicians alone would be to satisfy only a very small part of the requirement. Far more is needed. The nursing profession demands constant exploration of new knowledge. We need not only nurses who possess competence, compassion, and respect for the goals of society, but nurses who will become leaders in education and research.

Tyler suggests:

. . . [starting] the student from the beginning as an inquirer, as a person who is seeking to learn, giving [her] the skills and incentives that lead [her] to dig deeper into some sample of knowledge, and then encouraging [her] to go on independently while [she] is in school and in later life.*

* Tyler, *op. cit.*, p. 81.

We do not yet have all the answers. We must tell this to the student at the very outset. We must tell her that all the knowledge acquired in school is not to be construed as definitive; that *one does not learn, nor is it possible to learn all the answers for all time*. The student should be made aware that education must continue throughout a lifetime.

If we can build into educational programs the kinds of objectives that will encourage students to become lifelong inquirers, we can hope that significant progress will follow. We should tell our nursing school graduates that they are just entering upon the threshold of knowledge in nursing; that as graduating students they have achieved only the initial objectives of a program designed to prepare them to assume positions as team leaders. There are goals beyond these. Graduation from a school of nursing is not a point of completion, it is a point of continuation in an on-going program of professional development. If we succeed in conveying this concept, we may nurture and excite the minds of some nursing students to go on to make significant contributions to some of the problems that "plague" us today.

These then are the guidelines recommended by educators and psychologists to assist nursing educators in establishing objectives. The critical requirements approach is one way to achieve clarification of the broad, general goals proposed.

Bibliography

Cronbach, Lee J. *Educational Psychology*, Harcourt, Brace and Company, Inc., New York, 1954.

Dressel, Paul L. and associates. *Evaluation in Higher Education*, Houghton Mifflin Company, Boston, 1961.

Flanagan, John C. "The Critical-Requirements Approach to Educational Objectives," *School and Society*, 71:321-24, 1950.

Flanagan, John C. *et al. The American High School Student*, Houghton Mifflin Company, Boston, in press.

Gagné, Robert M. "Educational Objectives and Human Performance," chapter in *Learning and the Educational Process* by John Krumboltz, Rand McNally & Company, Chicago, 1965.

Krumboltz, John D. *Learning and the Educational Process*, Rand McNally & Company, Chicago, 1965.

Lindvall, C. M. *Defining Educational Objectives*, a report of the Regional Commission on Educational Coordination and the Learning Research and Development Center, University of Pittsburgh Press, 1964.

Mager, Robert F. *Preparing Objectives for Programmed Instruction*, Fearon Publishers, San Francisco, 1962.

Mager, Robert F., and McCann, Joseph. *Learner Controlled Instruction*. Varian Associates, Palo Alto, 1961.

O'Malley, Clair D. "Nursing in a Space-Age Hospital," *Am. J. Nursing*, 62: 54-58, (Dec.) 1962.

Tyler, Ralph W. "Some Persistent Questions on the Defining of Objectives," in *Defining Educational Objectives*, C. M. Lindvall (ed.), University of Pittsburgh Press, 1964.

Critical Incident

Miss Francis, the instructor in social problems in nursing, re-viewed the objectives of the course with the students at the initial class session. One of the objectives of her course was that the student would "conduct a conference utilizing the principles of group dynamics," before the completion of the course.

Miss Ward, an intermediate student, was observed conduct-ing a conference on the "preparation of the cardiac patient for the transition from the hospital to home care." Miss Ward had invited the public health coordinator to act as a consultant at the conference. Each student had been given a particular prob-lem, prepared by Miss Ward, to solve before presentation at the conference.

This is an effective critical incident. Miss Ward demon-strated outstanding leadership in her handling of the confer-ence and in inviting a consultant, knowledgeable in the specific field, to sit in on the conference as an advisor. Her presentation of specific problems to each member of the team indicated ad-vance preparation in anticipation of the conference. By assign-ing a problem to each participant she did an outstanding job of delegating responsibility to members of the nursing team.

Chapter 4
Using Critical
Incidents to
Define Behaviors

Meaningful objectives must be stated in behavioral terms. The identification and development of lists of critical behaviors for any activity require careful study of just what people do who are engaged in the activity. Once the behaviors are defined, it should be possible to set forth a list of objectives based on the critical requirements a person should possess to work in that field.

Before entering a discussion of the use of critical incidents to define behaviors for objectives in schools of nursing, it is appropriate to consider just what is meant by the term "objective."

WHAT IS AN EDUCATIONAL OBJECTIVE?
Mager states:

> An objective is an *intent* communicated by a statement describing a proposed change in a learner—a statement of what the learner is to be like when he has successfully completed a learning experience. It is a description of a pattern of behavior we want the learner to be able to demonstrate.*

An objective should be stated in terms of *the measurable change* in behavior that will be apparent and observable in the learner after completion of a unit or program of instruction.

After a demonstration by the student it should be possible for several qualified observers to reach agreement on the facts (1) that there has been a change in the behavior of the student, and (2) that the degree of change is acceptable in terms of the stated objectives.

* Robert F. Mager. *Preparing Objectives for Programmed Instruction*, Fearon Publishers, San Francisco, 1962, p. 3.

The committee on objectives and the faculty should decide *what is important*. Once this has been determined, broad, general goals should be refined in terms of the kinds of educational programs that will be appropriate for guiding students through every level of learning. Curriculum objectives and course objectives should be developed consistent with the over-all objectives of the school. To implement these objectives the faculty should develop lists of expected behaviors regarded as desirable outcomes.

FORMULATING STATEMENTS OF OBJECTIVES

Statements of objectives should be free of ambiguity, vagueness, or broad generalizations. Mager found that certain descriptive words are inappropriate.* He lists "words open to many interpretations" that should be avoided and "words open to fewer interpreations" that should be used.

Words open to many interpretations	*Words open to fewer interpretations*
To know	To write
To understand	To recite
To really understand	To identify
To appreciate	To differentiate
To fully appreciate	To solve
To grasp the significance of	To construct
To enjoy	To list
To believe	To compare
To have faith in	To contrast

(The two lists are not intended to be direct substitutions for one another; they are independent lists.)

Mager points out that it is seldom possible for two or more people to agree on exactly what is meant by "understanding," "appreciation," or "ability to grasp."† It is virtually impossible to measure what these terms mean without further clarification. Adding the word "really" does nothing to clarify the "understanding" and the word "fully" is equally vague. For example, in writing objectives for nursing education we should avoid statements such as:

Should be able to fully understand her responsibilities to her patient.

This is an inadequate statement; there is no definition of what is meant by "an understanding," and "responsibilities of a nurse" are not described. Does it mean the student should learn the principles of nursing care from books? Does it mean she should be aware of her legal obligations as a

---

* Mager, *op. cit.*, p. 11.
† Mager, *loc. cit.*

nurse? Does it mean she should "understand" in the sense that she can repeat codes of ethics from memory? Or, does it mean that she can quote and recite principles and also demonstrate behaviors appropriate for a professional nurse?

Cronbach indicates that there can be three different levels of *understanding*: (1) initial arbitrary associations that do not possess meaning, (2) ability to state principles and cite examples, (3) ability to judge validity by relating one principle to others in solving unfamiliar problems.*

Compare the general objectives cited above with the statements that follow:

> Upon graduation the student should possess the knowledge, attitudes, skills, and appreciation that will enable her to give safe, adequate, competent patient care as a general duty nurse in medical, obstetric, pediatric, psychiatric, and intensive care nursing, and to practice health teaching and home care in each of these areas.

At the course or instructional unit level:

> Given a list of basic principles relating to body mechanics, the student can demonstrate correct movements needed to shift a patient from the operating table to the cart.

> Given the assignment of caring for a patient that is being regulated on insulin, the student can assist in solving the problems concerned with diet and the establishment of electrolytic balance.

Statements such as these define the behaviors required of the student. If she can fulfill the requirements in each of these situations by demonstrating the desired behaviors, she can meet the objectives of at least two units of instruction.

Mager cautions that objectives should not be "worked over" until they demonstrate all the desired characteristics, but until they cover some aspect of the educational program as a whole or some important segment. Many statements may need to be written initially to cover broad objectives. All the desirable characteristics cannot be covered in every case, but each should include at least one of these points: (1) communication of intent, (2) definition of measurable change, or (3) establishment of standard of acceptability.

If objectives are developed in terms of these three requirements, it should be possible (1) to prepare statements to guide teachers and students, (2) to develop lists of measurable behaviors that should lead to the achievement of the objectives, (3) to establish standards of performance for completion of each course and for graduation from a particular school of

---

* Lee J. Cronbach, *Educational Psychology*, Harcourt, Brace and Company, Inc., New York, 1954, pp. 296-97.

nursing, and (4) to develop methods and procedures to measure and evaluate the changes in student behavior.

At each level of the education program the process of defining objectives becomes more specific; however, the basic characteristics remain the same. It is still necessary to communicate the *intent*, to identify the behaviors, and to establish standards of acceptability. This may become long and involved. There is bound to be disagreement; individuals disagree, schools disagree, and authorities often disagree. Some schools emphasize the patient-centered approach to teaching; others do not. Some include courses in communication, in physics, or in anthropology; others do not. These are just a few of the differences to be reconciled by the committee on objectives for a particular school.

DEFINING TERMINAL BEHAVIOR

The first level of agreement in formulating objectives is to decide on the *terminal behavior* to be demonstrated. *What kinds of care* should a graduate of this particular school be able to demonstrate? The final statement should be sufficiently clear and comprehensive that it identifies terminal behavior in a way that is readily understood at all levels from instructor to student—one that can be used not only as an end objective, but as a working statement.

Mager describes terminal behavior as the kind of *performance* expected upon completion of a program, course, or activity.* At our present state of knowledge, the only *observable* human behaviors are those that are overt and demonstrated by the things people do. This must be our starting point. We must use it as our basis for defining terminal behavior: descriptions of *observable performance* demonstrating degrees of change from beginning (or entering) behavior to ending (or terminal) behavior at the completion of a unit of instruction, a course, or a program.

The most important function of a statement of objectives is to provide explicit definitions of the *kinds of performance* or the *kinds of changes in behavior* to be demonstrated. With this in mind, examine the following statement:

> At the end of the course in integrated science the student should be capable of critical thinking.

On the surface this sounds good! It even sounds comprehensive. But, important though this may be in nursing, the statement tells nothing of the *measurable kinds of performance* the student should be able to demonstrate. How does one measure critical thinking? It is virtually impos-

* Mager, *op. cit.*, pp. 13-15.

sible. At present we can merely measure the outcomes of a student's thinking, and to do so we must have a standard.

Because of the difficulty in interpreting terms such as "critical thinking" and "understanding" we need more specific statements about student behavior. The following should be useful in describing desired behaviors in a given activity in nursing:

Example 1. Nursing Care of Diabetic Patients

After studying nursing care of the diabetic patient the student is expected to be able to:

1. Develop a nursing care plan consistent with the medical care plan.
2. Differentiate the symptoms of diabetic acidosis and insulin shock and initiate nursing measures for the prevention of both.
3. Do a urine reduction test and identify the degree of sugar content according to the color index.
4. Assist the patient to recognize dietary needs and follow his prescribed diet.
5. Instruct the patient in the proper care of skin, nails, and feet.
6. Initiate a plan to enable the patient to perform the following: self-injection of insulin, self-testing of urine, recognition of unusual symptoms.
7. . . . .

This list is comprehensive. It should enable teachers or observers of student performance (1) to reach agreement as to whether or not the student performs each of the steps; and (2) to determine whether or not that performance meets acceptable standards in the care of diabetic patients.

The key factor in the statement of objectives shown above is the identification of specific, observable behaviors required in the care of a diabetic patient. This list not only provides objectives, it also provides the basis for evaluating student performance. There should be little doubt about how to assess the performance of the intellectually gifted student who is merely able to recite the list and explain reasons why each step is necessary to good patient care, but who cannot give an injection or cannot communicate with the patient. An observer using the earlier statement of objectives might assume that this student is capable of "critical thinking" because she can discuss various aspects of the care of a diabetic patient. However, the observer who uses the second statement has more explicit information on which to evaluate the student. The specific behaviors to be observed include development of the nursing care plan, the initiation of preventive measures to avoid insulin shock, performance of urinalysis, and teaching the patient self-care. This type of description is useful to the teacher in teaching, and to the student in learning the care of a diabetic patient. It can also be useful for evaluating performance.

Example 2. Nursing Care of Patients in the Intensive Care Unit*

A student who meets the objectives in both theory and planned experience in Nursing Care of Patients in the Intensive Care Unit will be expected to do the following:

1. Describe the policies governing the admission of patients to the intensive care unit.
2. Identify the most common types of acute illness with emphasis on those that are prevalent in the intensive care area.
   a. Know which conditions generally cause acute illness.
   b. Know which conditions produce acute illness and can be expected in an industrial environment.
   c. Identify what types of acute illness can be expected in various geographical locations.
3. Identify patient problems that may occur during acute illness and make a sound nursing diagnosis.
   a. Gather pertinent facts related to patients.
   b. Identify the nursing care needs.
   c. Confer with physician on medical care plans.
4. Perform nursing skills under stress conditions.
   a. Apply basic nursing skills acquired in previous experiences.
   b. Know location of emergency equipment.
   c. Apply emergency nursing measures when indicated.
   d. Know and be able to operate monitoring devices.
   e. Know how to operate other new and improved equipment in use in the intensive care area.
   f. Use critical analytic approach in making nursing decisions in stress situations.
   g. Give comprehensive nursing care to an acutely ill patient.
5. Identify the significance of the emotional impact of acute illness on the patient and his family.
   a. Identify the emotional problems that may be anticipated in acute illness.
   b. Identify the effect of emotional strain on physical illness.
   c. Observe and report behavior changes that occur in the patient due to emotional strain.
   d. Establish rapport with patient and family.
   e. Identify the methods by which the nurse can assist emotionally disturbed patients and families to ease tension.
   f. Keep the family advised on patient's condition.
   g. Confer with the physician before advising family.

* The objectives of the course in this unit will depend upon the objectives of the department, types of patients admitted, and other factors. The sample has been developed as a guide and is not necessarily complete.

h. Arrange for conference between physician and family when necessary.

i. Know the value of permitting the family to visit briefly with the patient.

j. Assist the patient to adjust to the intensive care unit.

k. Assist the patient to recognize the value of expert nursing care during acute illness.

6. Identify the social and spiritual needs of the acutely ill patient.

a. Establish rapport with patient in order to communicate effectively.

b. Accept each patient as a unique individual with his own particular needs.

c. Identify social problems that may contribute to illness and subsequently produce physical changes.

d. Identify the social problems that can alter recovery.

e. Arrange for visitation of the social worker if need arises.

f. Identify the need for spiritual guidance during acute illness.

g. Know how to contact religious advisors of various faiths.

h. Arrange for visitation of clergyman if so indicated by the patient.

i. Tolerate and respect each patient's religious convictions.

j. Assist the patient to recognize his limitations during the acute stage of the illness and to recognize measures that will return him to an active normal life as his condition will permit.

7. Identify the contribution of other members of the health team in the care of the acutely ill patient.

a. Interpret patient needs to the physician.

b. Arrange for consultation and visitation of the dietitian if need arises.

c. Notify the inhalation therapy team and intravenous team when indicated.

d. Identify the need for other members of the health team or consultants.

e. Cooperate with all members of the health team.

8. Plan, administer, and evaluate a nursing care plan for an acutely ill patient.

a. Identify nursing functions.

b. Identify nursing procedures and activities to be emphasized.*

c. Identify typical and atypical nursing care to be given.

d. Execute the plan.

e. Utilize the nursing care plan for continuity of patient care.

f. Revise the nursing care plan consistent with patient's needs.

* Faye Abdellah, Irene Beland et al. Patient-Centered Approaches to Nursing. The Macmillan Company, New York, 1961, pp. 16-17.

g. Report pertinent facts to appropriate person.

h. Record accurate and descriptive findings on nurses' notes.

i. Implement the problem-solving technique in planning and giving nursing care.

USING CRITICAL INCIDENTS TO DESCRIBE BEHAVIORS

Statements of objectives are frequently summarized in one comprehensive statement: for example, the student should be capable of giving total care to diabetic patients. This is an acceptable statement provided everyone involved understands "total care" in the same way. Since there is often margin for several interpretations of this term, more explicit information is needed. The most effective statements of objectives include detailed explanations of all that is involved.

Numerous techniques may be used to describe behavior. For our purposes we will discuss two: the critical incident approach, and the performance analysis approach.

The *critical incident technique* has been widely used to identify behavioral requirements in many fields. Some of these were discussed in Chapter 2. The specific method is to gather facts of performance based on firsthand observations of nurses at all levels. It involves an intensive study of just what the nurse must do in all aspects of her work including application of technical knowledge and skills, the use of specific procedures, the development of a nursing diagnosis of patient needs, and the coordination of all activities with medical diagnosis and medical orders. In addition, facts should be gathered about the personality traits of the nurse, her ability to interact with other people, to communicate, to relate. All of this information is important in the development of descriptions of nursing behavior. Collecting critical incidents would be a very useful approach to the problem.

The *performance analysis approach* (sometimes called the task analysis approach) is another method that has been very useful in studying performance (described in Chapter 7). Here the emphasis is on detailed descriptions of the person, the equipment, the environment, and the other people involved in an activity. In this case, the term *task* refers to *any kind of systematic behavior*. At one end of the scale it could refer to the task involving the operation of a small device or piece of equipment, or the execution of a relatively simple procedure; at the other end it could refer to a complex process involving problem-solving, the application of critical thinking, and sound judgment.

Using the unit or task approach, performance descriptions can be developed that describe in detail all the interaction between people, equipment, or materials, and the environment within which they work.

SETTING ACCEPTABLE STANDARDS
OF PERFORMANCE

In any activity where performance is involved, we need minimum standards of acceptability. When equipment is used, and people must do certain things to cause the equipment to function, it is fairly easy to set minimum standards. There is a required set of steps the person must follow in order to get the equipment to operate. The outcomes can be described, and it is usually not too difficult to tell whether the result was satisfactory, or sufficient. For example, when an operator fails to press the appropriate button, or to shift a specific lever, the equipment does not function properly. If the equipment functioned on a partial basis, it may be possible to complete a cycle of work, but only so far. A minimum standard must be established so that it is possible to estimate the point at which the performance was not sufficient to complete the task in a satisfactory manner.

When no equipment is involved and performance is dependent upon the person behaving in some way to achieve results, it is somewhat more difficult to set the minimum standard unless outcomes are clear-cut. For example, there are many things a nurse can do to comfort a patient who is depressed about impending surgery; however, there are no clear-cut steps to be followed. Several combinations of behaviors could contribute to comforting the patient. Many variables are involved since no two patients are alike and seldom are two situations exactly alike. Here, the feelings of the patient must be identified, reasons for his fear must be considered, judgment is needed in making the decision about what to tell the patient. Setting minimum standards for successful behavior is considerably more difficult where covert problems are involved. The behavior required of the nurse may vary from simply listening to the patient discuss his condition, to the more complex behavior of identifying some of the patient's basic emotional needs, which are often manifest in a crisis.

In establishing standards of performance we must have a thorough knowledge of what should be done to complete an assignment and the kinds of behavior it requires. Where outcomes are not immediately evident, experience should provide the basis for including or excluding certain behaviors. In tasks or procedures, limits of time can be established together with a series of steps needed to do the work. Statements of minimum standards are needed before objective evaluation of performance can take place. These statements should be carefully developed and submitted for impartial tryout by other experienced people before they are put into use.

The development of statements of objectives involves (1) the identification of the desired terminal behavior, (2) detailed descriptions of the behaviors required to achieve the stated outcome, and (3) a set of standards of acceptability. If all three of these stipulations are met, it should be possible for committees to develop well-defined statements of objectives.

ORIENTING THE FACULTY
TO EDUCATIONAL OBJECTIVES

When the committee has resolved the matter of formulating the statements of objectives for a school, their work is not yet completed. There is more to be done. The statements must be submitted in written form to the faculty. Teachers should have an opportunity to study the statements.

The next step involves the development of the curriculum at each level consistent with the over-all objectives of the school. This is usually done by committees of educational administrators and teachers with relevant experience in certain fields. Curriculum development is meticulous work and must be an on-going process, particularly in a school of nursing where new knowledge and new techniques are emerging rapidly. Numerous experts have developed procedures for approaching the problem of developing the curriculum, but a great deal of research still is needed in this area. A brief discussion of curriculum development is presented in Chapter 5. Committees on curriculum development should be guided by the objectives of the school and use the best available sources of information about educational programs.

The third step is to develop course content consistent with the curriculum. Again, painstaking care is required to make the appropriate decisions about the inclusion and exclusion of certain materials. There are many new resources in education—textual materials, teaching methods, audiovisual aids, and other innovations. Decisions must be made about the kinds of learning experiences the students should have to reinforce what they learn from reading. Constant review and revision of course content and learning experiences are needed to make certain they are current and in keeping with the requirements of the curriculum.

The integration of learning experiences and course content is important in achieving the objectives of the curriculum. Success is dependent not only on effective guidelines in developing the course, but upon effective teaching, and effective evaluation of the results.

Where quantitative measures of progress are possible, it should be relatively easy to determine whether students are meeting the objectives. Achievement tests, written situation tests, or situational performance tests all yield evidence of accomplishment. If students do well on written tests, teachers have some evidence of a certain type of learning of the academic information presented. When students can demonstrate the application of what they have learned by giving acceptable patient care, teachers have evidence of the achievement of a measure of professional growth and development.

Orientation of the faculty involves (1) the presentation of the school objectives, (2) assistance in developing the curriculum at each level, (3) assistance in developing course content consistent with the objectives of the curriculum and the planning of relevant learning experiences, and (4) the establishment of effective methods for evaluating student performance and progress. Close cooperation is required to accomplish all these steps. Constant review and revision are needed to make certain that objectives are being accomplished in the most efficient manner and that the objectives fill the needs of the individual, the school, and society.

ORIENTING THE STUDENTS
TO EDUCATIONAL OBJECTIVES

Objectives are also important at the student level. They should not be regarded as the private property of the administrative body or the faculty. It is important that the students have access to this information. At the beginning of each course, and of every unit within the course, the teacher should take the time to explain what is to be accomplished and to define the goals to be met. Each student should be aware of just what is expected in the way of changes in her behavior, how the new information she learns will enhance her general store of knowledge, and how each unit of instruction relates to other units. Teachers should explain what each unit contributes to the over-all objectives of the course.

Three examples of instructional units are given together with explanations of their objectives.

Unit 1. Objective—To Insert a Foley Catheter

This is explained to the student at the outset of the unit of instruction following previous courses in anatomy and asepsis. The catheter is shown to the student, and its purposes are explained. The insertion of the catheter is demonstrated to the student, and each step is described in detail. Students are permitted to ask questions. These are answered. Criteria for correct insertion of the Foley catheter are discussed. Students then return the demonstration. After a given amount of practice, the student performs the insertion of the Foley catheter in actual practice in the clinical area. Her behavior is observed and checked by the instructor, who determines whether the student performed each of the steps required and how competently each step was accomplished. The instructor should be able to decide whether the student performed the procedure correctly on the basis of established standards. The student should also be able to evaluate her own performance in terms of the objective to be accomplished. If she had difficulty at any point, the student should be aware of this and review the steps necessary to overcome the difficulty or ask for help. When the catheter has been inserted and the patient is comfortable, the student should be aware that she has met the objective. Fine points of her performance can be discussed with the instructor who should take into consideration the time required, the sequence in which the steps were taken, the observation of aseptic techniques, and the correct positioning of the catheter.

Unit 2. Objective—Learning to Administer Oral Medication

The objective should be described to the student following an earlier series of lessons on the character and properties of the medications to be administered. The student should have learned to note contraindications, such as checking the pulse before giving digitalis, the use of Lugol's solution in juice, or the use of water with cough medicine. Then steps should be taken to give oral medication to a number of patients and to have the student return the demonstration. Students should be told that the objectives of this lesson cover only the administration of oral medication. Other types of medication require special skills and knowledges such as the administration of hypodermic, intramuscular, or intravenous medications.

Unit 3. Objective—Identifying and Solving Problems in the Emotional Care of a Hemiplegic Patient

The objective is explained to the student in terms of the implications of the hemiplegic condition with a full explanation of the nature of the incapacitation involved. There should be discussion of the types of mental and emotional reactions the patient may have, the obligations the patient has to himself and to his family, the need to enlist the cooperation of the family, the recognition of the possible social problems involved, the identification of the possible spiritual needs of the patient to help him understand and meet his problems, the effects of deprivation, strain, and worry, the development of a plan for convalescence.

In Unit 3, the outcomes are not immediate; it is considerably more difficult to teach this type of nursing care and to learn it. Each patient is different and accepts his incapacitation in a different way. The students may not always have an opportunity to observe examples of each kind of situation. Students must learn to generalize. There is also a need to bring together much that has been learned in courses in psychology, communication, and body care. There are no clear-cut, step-by-step procedures to be followed. The process is complex, and the tools are intangible. Achieving the objective of helping the patient to solve his emotional problems involves the use of good judgment and successful communication; estimates of the degree to which the objectives have been met must be made on the basis of an evaluation of the patient's adjustment to his situation, his acceptance of the problem, his emotional and mental outlook, and his attitude about the future. If the nurse has achieved the objectives, the patient should have a more positive outlook. The student cannot help him to cope with his problems, but she can help to show him how he can help himself.

Students who are aware of the objectives in a unit of instruction can understand what they must achieve and can proceed more systematically to accomplish their goals. Objectives can also serve as incentives to motivate students toward improving their behavior and toward achieving more than immediate outcomes.

Students who know what they are trying to achieve can evaluate their own progress in terms of expected behaviors and anticipated outcomes. Self-evaluation can be more effective when students understand how they should think, feel, and act as a result of learning something new and, most importantly, how to apply this new knowledge to patient care. Students who know the objectives of instruction can relate the new learning and achievement to their ultimate goal of becoming competent nurses.

KEEPING PACE WITH CHANGE

Committees on objectives should bear in mind that the formulation of objectives cannot be regarded as a one-time decision. Objectives cannot be fixed in point of time to apply from then on. Scientific, technical, and educational information is constantly changing, and new knowledge is emerging at a rapid rate. Thus it is constantly necessary not only to review and revise course content and the curriculum, but to review and revise school objectives to keep them current with the rapid pace of change.

Periodically the question must be posed: Are the objectives consistent with the needs of society, the school, the teacher, and the student? If licensing requirements become more stringent or if they change, educational objectives must be changed accordingly. As new teaching techniques become available, these should be used to achieve objectives. Keeping current implies the need for a committee to review, revise, and update objectives at all levels to cope with the changing requirements in nursing.

Bibliography

Cronbach, Lee J. *Educational Psychology*, Harcourt, Brace and Company, Inc., New York, 1954.

Krathwohl, David R. "Stating Objectives Appropriately for Program, for Curriculum and for Instructional Materials Developed," With the Researchers, *J. Teacher Education*, 16:83-92, (March) 1965.

Lindvall, C. M. (ed.). *Defining Educational Objectives*, a report of the Regional Commission on Educational Coordination and the Learning Research and Development Center, University of Pittsburgh Press, 1964.

Mager, Robert F. *Preparing Objectives for Programmed Instruction*, Fearon Publishers, San Francisco, 1962.

National League for Nursing. *Toward Excellence in Nursing Education*, The League, New York, 1964.

Critical Incident

Miss Older, an advanced-level student, was recently elected president of the student government association. At the first meeting following her election, she prepared an agenda using accepted parliamentary standards. Under "new business" she asked for volunteers to participate in a citywide poliomyelitis immunization campaign.

This is an effective critical incident. Two of the stated objectives of the school of nursing program in this school were (1) to make available opportunities for the development of both personal and professional growth and (2) to provide a channel for the development of initiative and self-direction in professional and civic affairs.

Miss Older in assuming the presidency of the student government association demonstrated willingness and capability to assume responsibility beyond class assignments. She reviewed parliamentary procedure and conducted the meeting in accordance with accepted practices. By initiating student participation on a voluntary basis in a communitywide immunization campaign, she demonstrated willingness to participate actively in constructive efforts toward improving the general health of the community. By seeking volunteers to assist in the campaign, she demonstrated self-direction and leadership.

Chapter 5

Developing Curriculum Objectives
and Learning Experiences
Consistent with Critical
Requirements in Nursing

One of the most difficult problems in the educational process is the development of the curriculum. A primary consideration is to build a curriculum to meet the needs of society, education, and the individual, with due consideration to prevailing philosophies, current theories of education, and the objectives of the school. Society and education serve each other interchangeably. Education provides the basis for increasing and expanding the scope of the individual, the family, and the society in which they function. Society within a community and a nation, on the other hand, makes certain demands on education to provide increasing background and capability to enable its people to function and endure within a complex and changing world.

WHAT IS THE PURPOSE
OF THE CURRICULUM?

A basic purpose of the curriculum in the school of nursing is to provide the educational experience and background to prepare the nurse in the technical competence needed to meet the demands of her profession. An additional requirement of an educational program is to provide the learning experiences that will enable the student to become a well-rounded, self-directed, competent nurse and individual, capable of participating actively and effectively as a member of her family, of her community, and of society. Therefore, the curriculum must be organized to provide learning experiences in each of the key areas: (1) professional, (2) personal and individual, (3) family, and (4) community and civic affairs.

Gardner tells us that the American way of life is unique in world societies.* Here performance is the primary determinant of status. Success

* John W. Gardner. *Excellence*, Harper & Brothers, New York, 1961, p. 123.

53

in any field of endeavor in our society is predicated on what the individual can do. If a student is highly motivated and has the academic ability and basic aptitudes for nursing, the school has an obligation to provide this student with an educational environment that will help her to achieve her full potential and to assume the responsibilities of her profession. Average achievement will not satisfy this type of student, therefore average educational opportunities will not suffice. The school of nursing should provide such a student with an educational background sufficiently rich in cultural, professional, and social learning experiences to prepare her for a stimulating career in nursing.

There have been a number of concepts about curriculum development and learning experiences and how these should be integrated to meet various needs. Some experts would eliminate subject matter in its formal sense in favor of an educational program that gives greater prominence to the needs of the student and the patient. These educators contend that subject matter should be integrated into broad aspects of the educational program, not in the formal way, but as adjuncts to the projects and activities in which the student engages. However, there is a solid segment of educators who still regard the inclusion of subject matter in the curriculum as a functioning factor. Others hold with the development of the activity-centered curriculum, and still others cling to a core curriculum. There are many mutations of these concepts.

It is the responsibility of the committee on curriculum development in each school to establish the kind of curriculum that will best fit that particular institution from the standpoint of the philosophy of the school, prevailing educational theories, the needs of society, and the needs of the individual student. It would be desirable to develop the curriculum on the basis of a systematic study of the critical requirements for success in nursing. Such a study would serve to identify the specific skills and knowledges needed along with other behavioral traits.

SELECTION AND ORGANIZATION
OF LEARNING EXPERIENCES

Learning is the keystone of education. It can be defined as a series of persistent changes resulting from actual experience rather than mere maturation.* Curriculum planning in a school of nursing should involve the selection of the kinds of learning experiences that will contribute both directly and indirectly to the academic and professional growth of the student and increase her capability to give competent patient care.

Brown identifies two kinds of preparation essential to the development

* Ole Sand and Helen Belcher. *An Experience in Basic Nursing Education*, G.P. Putnam's Sons, New York, 1958, p. 33.

of the competent nurse:* (1) higher education leading to professional growth in areas of problem-solving, including capability to collect pertinent information, to formulate and test hypotheses, to draw inferences and make conclusions based on findings, and to apply appropriate principles and theories in solving nursing problems; (2) technical preparation in professional practice to promote capability not only in the care of hospitalized patients, but in recognizing and assisting in the solution of problems involved in meeting the health needs of the community.

The Purpose of Learning Experiences

A recent publication from the National League for Nursing describes the function of learning experiences as follows:

> Learning experiences, carefully selected to show the relationship between classroom, clinical laboratory, and clinical nursing conferences, assist and guide the student by (1) stimulating independent thinking; (2) promoting the development of problem-solving skills; (3) pointing out the relationship of knowledge to its application in clinical nursing situations; (4) helping to increase depth and breadth of understanding; (5) stimulating the development of essential skills; and (6) encouraging intellectual and professional growth.†

Events in life often occur with an unstructured sequence. That is to say, although it is possible to prepare oneself through education and personal planning for favorable experiences in life, an individual cannot "guarantee" or even be reasonably sure of the events and situations he must face, because he cannot always be implicated directly in the selection of his experiences.

In education, a different situation prevails. It is possible for instructors to select and provide the kinds of learning experiences in which their students can participate. The higher the level of perception, sensitivity, and ability of the teacher or the curriculum planner, the more favorable the learning experiences for the student. The approach to teaching, the selection, the planning, and the manner of presentation of educational experiences can have important implications for student learning. These are the teacher activities in education.

However, it must be pointed out that regardless of the quality and caliber of the educational planning and the manner of teaching, something more is needed. The student and her state of readiness must also be considered. Educational experiences can have varying degrees of effectiveness and impact upon the student depending upon her preparation, motivation, and readiness to participate. Application, attitude, motivation, and resolution to persist are the important student activities in education.

* Esther Lucille Brown. *Nursing for the Future*, Russell Sage Foundation, New York, 1948, pp. 138-39.
† *Toward Excellence in Nursing Education*, National League for Nursing, New York, 1964, pp. 20-21.

Brown describes two levels of educational experience which are developed on the basis of the preparation of the student in point of time and sequencing of opportunities "which are student-centered from the standpoint of teaching, and patient-centered from the standpoint of learning:"*

First-Level Experiences
1. Emphasis on the need for sound evaluation of the patient's problems beginning with his initial visit to the doctor's office, and including psychogenic factors, nutritional factors, and a general investigation of all patient problems.
2. Discussion and identification of the patient's emotional involvement and trauma in facing impending surgery. Also an investigation of various means for alleviating some of this strain.
3. Demonstrations and discussions of bedside care emphasizing the importance of accurate observing and recording of patient signs and conditions.
4. Practice in helping patients to meet problems of facing relatively minor or simple surgical procedures.

Second-Level Experiences
1. Demonstration of and practice in developing nursing care plans and nursing diagnoses consistent with medical diagnoses. Practice in giving patient-centered care in anticipation of major surgery.
2. Practice in recall of information and knowledge appropriate to care of the patient facing major surgery and an ability to recognize problems and identify appropriate steps needed to provide competent, patient-centered care. Reinforcement of ability to think logically and act promptly to meet patient needs.
3. Demonstrations of and practice in assisting the patient to help himself in facing and solving some of his problems, both preoperatively and postoperatively. Practice in helping to prepare the patient to meet family and social problems which he will encounter and how he can rehabilitate himself to return to being a productive and participating member of society. Ability to recognize the degree and amount of guidance appropriate in such situations is important here.
4. Demonstrations of and practice in teaching health habits to the patient and to his family to develop more positive attitudes about general good health.†

The above list is focused primarily on nursing in the medical-surgical clinical situation. Some aspects of these experiences can be generalized to other areas of nursing education.

* Brown, *op. cit.*
† Amy Frances Brown. *Curriculum Development*, W.B. Saunders Company, Philadelphia, 1961, p. 586.

It should be re-emphasized that learning experiences such as those described above must be presented in a sequence appropriate to the level of learning the student has achieved. They should also be planned in a way to provide continuity from earlier experiences involving the application of theories, principles, and techniques. Continuity and sequencing in turn provide the basis for student integration of the learning experiences into her general body of knowledge.

Criteria for Selecting Learning Experiences

Tyler suggests a number of criteria for selecting appropriate learning experiences for nursing students. These were made in connection with the University of Washington Project on which Dr. Tyler served as a consultant.*

1. What opportunities does the experience provide for the learner to practice the kinds of behavior implied by the objective?
2. What opportunities does the learning experience give the learner to deal with the kinds of content implied by the objective?
3. What evidence is there that the student is obtaining satisfaction from the experience?
4. Is the reaction desired in the experience within the range of possibility for the students involved?
5. Is the experience appropriate to the student's present attainment, her predispositions, and the like?
6. What kinds of experiences have been developed, capitalizing on the various interests of both students and faculty members?
7. How is the experience related to the student's own purposes?
8. How does the experience provide an opportunity for the student to attain more than one objective?
9. Are undesirable outcomes avoided?

Tyler's criteria should be most useful to educational administrators and members of faculties as a basis for selecting learning experiences for curriculums in schools of nursing. As the curriculum is developed, consideration should be given to the value of each course in relation to the other courses and in relation to the academic and professional development of the student.

Sand and Belcher describe the importance of vertical and horizontal relationships between learning experiences. Vertical relationships are defined as those that broaden and deepen the student's knowledge and capability without undue repetition; whereas horizontal relationships are those that exist among the learning experiences a student has at a particular time

* Sand and Belcher, *op. cit.* Criteria formulated by Ralph W. Tyler for the University of Washington Project, pp. 79-80.

and the way in which various experiences tend to build upon, depend upon, and reinforce one another.*

There are numerous methods for achieving the vertical and horizontal relationships which produce the tapestry of learning. Dressel describes the use of logical order such as the presentation of historical events; moving from the simple to the complex as in teaching mathematical concepts and principles; moving from the specific to the general; beginning with the immediate and moving toward the remote, or generalizing from past to present.† All of these approaches can be useful in presenting educational experiences.

Relationships of courses in nursing schools have been achieved in many ways. In some schools students have been given courses in art, not art appreciation alone, but they are given opportunities to work in modeling clay or to paint. Courses of this type have been known to be effective in developing a sense of creativity and beauty, but to go a step beyond this, such learning experiences have also been instrumental in developing desirable concepts, values, and attitudes toward life. These can be generalized to embrace attitudes toward the nursing profession and toward people in general. In many schools there are courses in English composition and public speaking. What can these contribute to nursing? It has been found that communication skills are vital to success in nursing. Nurse-patient relationships depend upon effective communication skills. These skills can be developed through courses in writing, opportunities for discussion, and activities involving the organization of thoughts and ideas. Some nursing students take courses in physical education. The purpose of this type of learning experience is to develop good body mechanics and general physical fitness. In addition, sociology, psychology, and many other courses can help to provide the well-rounded educational and learning experiences needed in nursing.

Continuity, Sequencing, and Integration of Learning Experiences

In order to be of maximum benefit to student development, learning experiences should be presented within some meaningful framework. There is importance in continuity, for example. Isolated courses or fragments of learning experiences do little or nothing to contribute toward the development of the student. Often they are lost or forgotten soon after the experience ends. There must be a pattern of continuity whereby information and experiences are presented in a logical fashion both from the standpoint of information and the point in time in which they are presented. This does not imply that what is needed is constant repetition or review. This type of exercise can become deadly dull since the student receives little reinforce-

---

* Sand and Belcher, *op. cit.*, p. 43.
† Paul L. Dressel and associates. *Evaluation in Higher Education*, Houghton Mifflin Company, Boston, 1961, p. 15.

ment of the reason for the review. For example, mechanically practicing the reading of a scale from a series of illustrations has little meaning to the student. It is much more meaningful and reinforcing if the student first learns to read a scale from printed directions and is then asked to read scales using a manometer or a thermometer. Moving from theory to practice in any type of learning can provide valuable reinforcement. Learning about salts and acids is a matter of rote memorization if the student learns this information from a chemistry book and has no opportunity to apply it. However, when the student is given an opportunity to do an exercise involving urine reduction, she will have an occasion to apply her new knowledge in testing for sugar and acetone.

Continuity and sequencing of learning experiences help the student to use and apply new knowledge and to renew earlier experiences. Review and repetition in this sense permit the student to build from one experience to another. The matter of planned sequencing of units and phases of instruction is an important aspect of teaching. Cumulative learning experiences provide opportunities for the student to test her store of information, calling forth various skills and knowledges as needed. In this way it is possible to achieve integration in learning—relating present learning experiences directly or indirectly to past experiences both in and out of school. This implies making the learning experiences an integral part of the student's body of knowledge.

Critical incident studies can provide the list of behaviors to be included as part of learning experiences.

The two examples of learning experiences included here emphasize vertical and horizontal relationships and indicate evidence of continuity and sequencing of information. It is not assumed that these are presented as the only method for achieving such relationships, but rather as suggestions in the broad, general sense of the word.

Note in particular the list of observable behaviors. These are behaviors that can be verified if they take place at a time before the point at which the observer begins to note student activity.

Learning Experience I: Communication and Nurse-Patient Relationship

OBJECTIVE

To increase and improve ability to communicate with patients and to prepare them emotionally for impending surgery for craniotomy.

Prior learning experiences: courses in sociology and social problems in human behavior, psychology, communication skills, and other courses providing a background of scientific information.

Situation for learning includes: opportunity for review and recall, consultation visits, diagnostic tests, physical examination findings, doctor's progress notes, patient and family history and background, nurse's notes and nursing care plans. Nurse has opportunities for conversation with the patient regarding his attitude about being hospitalized and about his illness, and the fact that surgery is indicated.

Preparation for assignment to brief patient about impending surgery should involve review of the above information, recall of appropriate learning experiences about the nature of the surgery the patient will receive, and something about postoperative care in this type of situation. With this background in mind the nurse then prepares her nursing plan.

Nursing plan for briefing patient preoperatively for craniotomy:

1. Scheduled time for surgery announced to patient
2. Notified family
3. Explanation of shave preparation procedure
4. Reassurance of patient of the competence of the surgeon
5. Explanation of preoperative medications
6. Assurance of the skilled nursing care immediately available to him following surgery
7. Assurance that he will remain in the intensive care unit until the decision is made to return him to his room, the decision contingent upon his progress

One of the most important learning experiences for nursing students is in the area of changing attitudes toward other people and different ways of doing things. In nursing more than in any other profession the problem of interaction with people is a major factor. A nurse must administer to the needs of others to a far greater extent than in any other human interaction in the normal course of events. Business contacts, social situations, and other types of exchange are relatively casual by comparison.

Learning experiences planned in the area of changing attitudes should enable the student to learn to interact successfully with others in the nursing situation, with peers, with subordinates, with superiors, with the patient, and with the patient's family.

The following is an example of the general approach to the planning of a learning experience involving attempts to change some basic attitudes. In this case, ideal behaviors are listed along with less desirable ones. In a learning experience of this kind there is no clear-cut demonstration of a procedure, but rather it is necessary for the instructor to introduce appropriate comments and point out specific things as field trips proceed. At the end of a trip to one of the organizations mentioned, the class should take time to discuss the desirable behaviors again.

Discussion: Preliminary Preparation for Learning Experience II

Maier suggests that role playing is an effective method for teaching students various kinds of human relationships. He lists the behaviors regarded as essential:

1. A respect for other people
2. A belief that whatever people do or feel has been caused
3. A true feeling that people have needs which may not correspond to our own
4. A realization that perhaps all problems with people are matters of misunderstandings
5. An ability to see the frustrated individual not as bad, but as in need of understanding and help
6. A tolerance for people who may have less ability than others, but whose feelings may easily be hurt
7. A true feeling for the fact that everyone in a healthy state of mind wants to be a member of society and do a constructive job*

To these the authors would like to add

8. A realization that those who are ill or incapacitated are frequently in a depressed state of mind and in need of even more understanding and help than people who are in good health

Maier goes on to say that attitudes such as those listed above should replace the conflicting kinds of attitudes which are prevalent, but which should be overcome, such as:

1. The inclination to blame someone as a method of correction
2. The tendency to overlook the contribution of the situation to behavior and to see the individual as the only factor in behavior
3. The belief that fear motivation is basically sound
4. The belief that people want to do as little for as much as they can
5. The belief that kindness is a sign of weakness†

Learning Experience II. Changing Basic Attitudes

Building on the two sets of attitudes presented above, learning experiences can be planned in which the student takes alternate roles first as the patient, and later as the nurse. This type of experience offers excellent opportunities to develop the basic attitudes represented in the first list as opposed to attitudes of hostility, suspicion, and intolerance. In reversing roles it is possible for the student to experience the effects of hostile and aggressive treatment.

Another distinct advantage to role playing can be that of bringing about a change in the student's attitude toward herself. In the profession of nursing as in all other professions, a healthy self-concept is vitally important. Feelings of fear of failure, inadequacy, and the lack of confidence must be overcome. Learning experiences which enable the student to reduce or eliminate these problems can be very helpful.

Appropriate attitudes can be introduced into learning situations not

---

* Norman R. F. Maier. *Principles of Human Relations*, John Wiley & Sons, Inc., New York, 1952, p. 95.
† Maier, *loc. cit.*

only in role playing but in actual contacts with the patients and others on the staff.

The following activities can also provide meaningful examples of learning experiences which can be helpful in changing basic attitudes:

1. Selected field observation visits consistent with course content. Visits to rehabilitation centers, mental hospitals, health clinics
2. Lectures by visiting consultants from specialized fields, e.g., experts in lip reading, representatives from the school for the blind
3. Home care visits following hospitalization
4. Participation in student government committees and affairs
5. Participation in community activities involving health and welfare as well as civic affairs

An important factor in planning learning experiences for students in schools of nursing is to consider the kinds of satisfaction the students derive from the learning situations. A number of studies have shown that increased learning results when students experience a sense of satisfaction or self-fulfillment as a result of taking certain courses and in achieving certain objectives. Careful planning of learning experiences can help to encourage positive attitudes, appreciation, and appropriate professional behavior. When students are guided through enriched learning experiences, they can derive an increased appreciation for cultural values, for their profession, and for their roles as citizens in our society. When these basic objectives of education are achieved, they should persist and contribute to capability for self-direction.

IMPROVING THE LEARNING SITUATION

Goals and objectives in any educational program are significant only if the efforts of teachers and students alike are focused on activities designed to achieve the stated goals. Numerous approaches have been successful. These vary from the disease- and procedure-centered approaches to the more comprehensive problem-solving and patient-centered care approaches.

The Problem-Solving Approach to Patient-Centered Care

Only one of the various approaches to patient care will be presented—that of problem-solving in patient-centered care. In this approach there have been two schools of thought: (1) to study basic problems in nursing first and then to locate patients with these problems and endeavor to apply the theoretical knowledges and principles learned earlier; (2) to select a patient for whom a nursing diagnosis is available and to identify the problems involved and to proceed toward their solution.

Abdellah *et al.* identify two major classes of problems in patient-centered care: (1) the overt problems—those that are apparent and that both the patient and his family must face; and (2) the covert problems— those involving the intangible aspects of illness including anxieties, emotions, and fears. The nurse can assist in solving both types of problems, although the second group of problems mentioned requires greater depth and different skills. Some of the steps that Abdellah and her associates suggest in the use of problem-solving techniques are as follows:*

1. *Getting to know the patient.* This is a matter of establishing rapport and gaining the confidence of the patient to a sufficient degree that communication is established. Process recording could be utilized to enhance the interviewing skills of the student to facilitate communication. "The climate the nurse creates within the patient-nurse interaction influences the substance of the interview."† Bermosk and Mordan stress the fact that interviewing is both an art and a skill which the nurse should endeavor to develop for purposes of (1) obtaining information, (2) giving or sharing information, (3) allowing for the expression of feelings, (4) identifying and clarifying needs and goals, (5) teaching, and (6) counseling.‡

2. *Sorting out the facts and data about the patient.* The nurse has a number of sources of information about the patient: information about his physical state and symptoms, something of his background, information about his work, his family, and his medical history. In addition, facts can be gathered by interviewing the patient. From this information the nurse must sort out important details—those most relevant to the nursing situation—and develop her plan accordingly.

3. *Making generalizations about patient problems.* This involves making hypotheses about the situation. Experience with previous patients who had similar problems should enable the nurse to make some initial generalizations about the patient and his problems. However, the nurse should be extremely careful not to overgeneralize. It is important to remember that each patient has his own set of problems, and that there are sufficient variables in the situation to prevent using general rules for every patient.

4. *Verifying the patient's concept of his problems.* Patients differ markedly in their acceptance of illness and their need for nursing care. Some regard their problems realistically, others are caught in emotional binds that prevent them from viewing the situation objectively. It is important to verify the patient's concept of his problems and to help him to gain greater insight into the particular circumstance in which he finds himself. Often this in itself can do a great deal to stabilize the patient.

* Faye G. Abdellah. "Methods of Identifying Covert Aspects of Nursing Procedures," *Nursing Research*, 6:4, (June) 1947.
  † Faye G. Abdellah, Irene L. Beland, Almeda Martin, and Ruth V. Matheney. *Patient-Centered Approaches to Nursing*, The Macmillan Company, New York, 1961, p. 13.
  ‡ Loretta Sue Bermosk and Mary Jane Mordan. *Interviewing in Nursing*, The Macmillan Company, New York, 1964, p. 39.

5. *Deciding on therapeutic plans.* An important part of nursing is the development of a nursing care plan to fit the needs of each individual patient. The nurse must make a good nursing diagnosis and must develop a nursing care plan consistent with the medical care plan.

6. *Determining family attitudes about the patient's illness and enlisting their cooperation and assistance.* Often a nursing care plan may involve activities that are unfamiliar to the patient and to his family. It is important to discuss certain aspects of nursing care with the patient's immediate family to gain their support and approval. They, in turn, can often assure the patient that the procedures are necessary and that the nursing care should be helpful. Frequently the success of nursing care is contingent upon the cooperation and approval of the patient's family, who tend to reinforce the patient.

7. *Observing significant signs and symptoms in the patient's physical and emotional state.* The nurse must constantly be alert to all the significant signs and symptoms the patient may develop. At times these may be minute and difficult to discern. This is particularly true of the subtle changes in mood or other covert problems that may influence patient welfare.

8. *Recognition of interrelationship between the patient and the nurse.* At various stages of illness, the attitude of the patient may undergo a series of changes. There can be a shift from complete confidence and dependence to one of doubt and questioning of authority. The nurse should endeavor to maintain a continuing, harmonious relationship with the patient. Frequent review of patient progress and new problems that evolve during illness can help to keep the relationship a pleasant one.

9. *Modifying the nursing care plan to meet the patient's changing needs.* The complexity of the human body and its physical and emotional balance challenge the nurse to make constant adjustments in her nursing care plan to cope with each change. The problems of convalescence differ from those in the intensive care unit. One set of problems may give way to another within a matter of a few days. For this reason, there must be a great deal of flexibility in nursing care plans to allow for such contingencies and change. An alert nurse will make modifications as needed and will discuss with the patient the changes being planned, pointing out the benefits which will accrue to the patient from the change.

Problem-solving requires that the nurse exercise more than the fundamental skills and knowledges she has acquired. According to Abdellah and her associates, there are five basic elements in the problem-solving approach to patient care:

1. Mastery of technical and managerial skills
2. Ability to observe and report
3. Ability to interpret significant signs and symptoms
4. Ability to analyze nursing problems
5. Organizing plans and efforts to achieve objectives*

* Abdellah, *op. cit.,* p. 26.

The design and selection of learning experiences that emphasize these skills in relation to the foregoing steps should help to reinforce student learning. In addition to opportunities for use of specific knowledges and skills, the problem-solving approach provides excellent occasions for developing the attitudes and appreciations essential to competent patient-centered care.

Learning experiences in the identification and solution of nursing problems can be included in the curriculum in a variety of ways: by demonstration in bedside care, through written situation tests, in classroom discussion, and in actual patient contact under supervision. The important point to remember is that each nursing situation presents its own set of problems and that each opportunity helps the student to develop her powers of inductive and deductive reasoning.

TEACHER ACTIVITIES
IN THE LEARNING SITUATION

Much of the success in developing the climate and conditions for learning is dependent upon the approach to teaching. One set of teaching principles will not suit every learning situation; each requires special consideration concerning the appropriate information and content, the tools to be used, and the method.

Although teaching cannot be a fixed procedure, some functions are inherent in every teaching situation. Gagné states these include:*

1. *Presenting stimuli.* The presentation of appropriate stimuli, cues, or signals serves to initiate a response from the student. Much can be done with audiovisual aids, films, or television. Demonstrations in the laboratory can also serve to provide appropriate stimuli. For example, if a motor response is required, the instructor must present the kind of signal or cue that will initiate a motor response. If the student is required to adjust the weights on traction, she must be shown what to do and must be given an opporunity to practice. She should then be asked to adjust the weights. If a verbal response is required, the action may be initiated by asking a question: "Can you describe the brain and the spinal cord?" or "Can you identify four methods a physician can use to do a physical examination?"

2. *Directing attention.* This involves narrowing the field of possible responses the student might make by using key words or by actually physically pointing to an object. If several objects are involved in a demonstration, the teacher can direct attention to a specific object by placing it in front or above the others, or by pointing to it. If verbal clues are appropriate, the instructor can direct the student's thinking by saying something like the following: "Yesterday we studied the circulatory system and its

* Laurence Siegel. *Contemporary Theories of Instruction*, Chapter 3, "Instruction and the Conditions of Learning," by Robert M. Gagné, Chandler Publishing Company, San Francisco, 1965.

function." This will help to direct the student's thoughts to the topic to be discussed. Given this direction, she should begin to recall the discussion about the circulatory system.

3. *Describing objectives.* Moving from step 2, after the student has made the appropriate response, the instructor should state the objectives of the current lesson. Students tend to become more interested if they are given a description of an objective or a goal. In this case, the instructor might say: "Today we are going to discuss the properties and functions of the blood." The student will then be able to build on the basis of what she learned earlier about the circulatory system. Today's lesson should help her to understand the functions and properties of the blood. A great deal can be accomplished if the teacher takes the time to make a clear statement of the objective of the lesson—the reason this particular material is being discussed.

4. *Stimulating recall.* It is possible to help "trigger" recall of earlier learning by drawing from the student responses to relevant questions. For example, "Describe the circulatory system." Or, one could ask: "Do you remember in yesterday's lesson we discussed the circulatory system?" Both of these instructor activities can be used to stimulate recall of earlier experiences.

5. *Sequencing information.* The first four steps mentioned above should follow in the sequence presented: (1) presenting stimuli, (2) directing attention, (3) stating objectives, and (4) stimulating recall. The fifth step is contingent upon the nature of the responses the instructor is able to elicit by the four previous steps. The fifth step should be the appropiate "next" step to be taken in relation to the responses to the preceding steps. The fifth step can be chosen in a variety of ways. If the students demonstrate satisfactory recall of previous information and appear ready to take the next step, a new concept may be introduced. The size of the step can be determined by the quality of the response and what kind of learning has gone on before this lesson.

Readiness of the class is usually the basis for deciding when new learning experiences should begin; however, this may tend to penalize certain slow learners in the class. Assuming the decision is made that the class is ready to move on to the next step, a new lesson is presented. After a learning experience about the circulatory system, the blood and its functions, a next lesson might concern common diseases of the blood and the discussion might center around the effects of such diseases on arterial and venous circulation. The decision to review earlier lessons should be made if the students were unable to give a comprehensive description of the circulatory system and its functions.

6. *Guiding responses.* Sometimes information the student has been presented may not quite have "jelled," so to speak, and it may be necessary to provide a few extra clues to elicit the appropriate response. The in-

structor should recognize when this is necessary and should offer a leading question that will help pinpoint the problem for the student and help her to verbalize her thoughts and give the correct response. This can be done if some learning has taken place.

Another method for guiding student responses can help the student to experience one of the greatest thrills in learning—"discovering" something. Opportunities can be increased if the instructor can guide the student's thinking. For example, assuming no prior knowledge of the circulatory system had been acquired, it is possible to create a "moment of discovery" for some alert student by asking a question such as: "One of the functions of the circulatory system is to provide and maintain the flow of oxygen to the body; how do you think this is achieved?" In this way the student is guided toward "discovery" of some way whereby the need for the flow of oxygenated blood to the body and the removal of deoxygenated blood from the system can be established, and this will lead to readiness for learning the next system, the respiratory system.

7. *Promoting generalization.* Increased learning can be achieved when the student conceives possibilities for the application of a concept or a principle to some new situation. The instructor should try to provide opportunities for students to make such generalizations. For example, when the student learns that body tissue damage results when there is a sustained lack of oxygen, she should be able to make the generalization that there probably would be a possibility of brain damage in an instance where a small boy was buried for several hours in a rockslide.

8. *Evaluating progress.* Information is returned to both student and teacher at this point: (1) To the student through evaluations of the quality of her work and the responses she makes, e.g., the instructor gives the student an evaluation of a return demonstration of the effects on the patient when traction is increased. If the student can describe the purpose of adjusting the weights and the scientific principle involved, the instructor should advise the student that her performance has been effective. (2) To the teacher, there is feedback in the form of deductions that can be made on the adequacy of the responses the students make. When responses are inadequate, the problem may not always be a matter of the student's failure to understand. Sometimes, there is need for revision in the method of presentation, or a need for review, re-emphasizing certain aspects of the lesson.

Regardless of the approach, teacher activities involve the eight functions described. Implicit in each of these steps, of course, is the appropriate use of teaching tools. Dressel identifies some of the many instruments available for increasing the effectiveness of teaching.*

* Paul L. Dressel and associates. *Evaluation in Higher Education,* Houghton Mifflin Company, Boston, 1961, p. 14.

1. Educational materials (books, including textbooks and supplemental books), required or optional reading materials, current periodicals, teaching machines, syllabuses, slides, films, tapes, recordings, television.
2. Improved instructional methods (lectures, discussion, demonstrations, situational problems, case problems involving actual experience with patients, individual conferences, seminars, guest speakers, audiovisual aids including programed learning techniques)
3. Relevant outside assignments (reading, problems, papers, oral reports)
4. School and extracurricular activities (laboratory, observation, internships, actual nursing experience on tours of duty, travel, lectures, continued reading in the field)
5. Effective evaluation methods (objective tests, situational performance tests, essays, papers, reports, class participation, peer judgment, self-evaluation, observations of performance by instructors and others qualified in nursing)

Tools alone cannot "make the critical difference" in teaching. Preliminary preparation on the part of the teacher is required if students are to be presented with learning experiences that will be important and meaningful. Some suggested approaches to the preparation of materials are presented in the following section.

Guide to the Preparation of Instructional Materials

Miller proposes several steps to guide teacher preparation of instructional materials. Careful preparation can do much to provide conditions conducive to learning.*

1. *Prepare an outline* based on a description of what the student is suppose to be able to do as a result of learning the new information.
2. *Break the information down into small segments or phases of instruction.*
3. *Describe what the student will learn in each unit.*
4. *Describe the instruments, materials, or equipment involved.*
5. *Make plans for evaluation of progress.*

This approach may be used in teaching not only fundamental nursing skills but also various aspects of patient-centered care as well.

Acceptance of the responsibility for teaching imposes stringent demands on those who plan the instructional program. An important factor in the teaching situation is the *student*. Students are not just a group; they are

* Robert B. Miller. A *Suggested Guide to Functional Characteristics of Training and Training Equipment*, Technical Memorandum ML-TM-56-14. Maintenance Laboratory, Air Force Personnel and Training Research Center, Air Research and Development Command, Lowry Air Force Base, Colorado, May, 1956, pp. 32-33.

individuals and, as such, they require consideration of the kinds of individual differences that exist in background, personality, aptitude and ability, readiness for learning, and motivation. Some of the problems in coping with individual differences are presented in the following section.

Recognizing Individual Differences

Marked differences between individual students in any educational program present a challenge to the instructor. In a national survey of aptitudes and abilities of high-school students (440,000) it was found that some students can learn certain kinds of information at nearly twice the rate of others. This same study revealed that between 20 and 30 per cent of the students in the ninth grade in high school knew more about a number of subject-matter fields than the average twelfth-grade student.*

These are just a few of the kinds of individual differences that can exist among students in any type of school. In a school of nursing, it can mean that some students in the class will bring to the learning situation a background in which there were opportunities for cultural development and enriched programs of education, whereas others may come to the classroom situation lacking even the basic prerequisites. Some of the problems are reduced through the screening process; however, wide differences still exist, and other differences tend to develop as students participate in new learning experiences. Some will readily adapt to learning nursing fundamentals; others may be able to learn the theoretical aspects of nursing but lack the ability to practice nursing at the bedside.

Teaching in the classroom situation often requires that the teacher present instructional materials at the level of the average student. This means a penalty is imposed on the students at either extreme. The more advanced students are handicapped because they are required to reduce their normal pace of learning to match that of the average student. The slower students are handicapped because the pace is too fast and they find it difficult to keep up with the class.

New educational methods and media have been developed to overcome some of these problems. Individualized instruction is an innovation in teaching that makes it possible for each student to learn at a rate commensurate with her own capability. When students are permitted to undertake new material at the point when they are ready to learn it, motivation to learn tends to be much greater. When the student is ready, she need not wait for the others in the class to reach her point of readiness, she may proceed to the next lesson without delay; she feels rewarded and encouraged to continue. On the other hand, in the case of the slow learner,

* John C. Flanagan, Frederick B. Davis, John T. Dailey, Marion F. Shaycoft, David B. Orr, Isadore Goldberg, Clinton A. Neyman, Jr. *The American High School Student*, University of Pittsburgh, 1964 (in press at Houghton Mifflin Company, Boston, in 1966) p. 14-2 in preliminary printing.

there is less chance of frustration because the student is at liberty to review and take her time until she does learn and is ready for the next step. The slow student is not made to feel inferior because she cannot keep pace, nor does she lose out because the instructor and the class move on and she cannot understand the discussion.

Individualized instruction is still relatively new and much more research is needed; however, a great deal has already been done. Klaus states that autoinstruction

... promotes the orderly and controlled development of an individual's skill in much the same way as a good tutor might do. By presenting lessons in small, carefully sequenced steps, complicated skills can be developed by gradually progressing from very simple to very complex levels of performance . . . the autoinstructional technique facilitates the evaluation and improvement of the materials during the course of their development in that the difficulty level of contribution of each step can be carefully ascertained and, when necessary, any step may be modified or revised.*

In the field of nursing education a great deal can be taught through the use of autoinstructional materials. Several researchers have already conducted studies to determine the relative merits of using this approach, and many more are being published. One of the earliest studies was conducted by Seedor and presented as an "Introduction to Asepsis."† The author described her work in developing the program for teaching asepsis and its evaluation in a later report.‡ Crayton and Lysaught prepared "An Introduction to Radiation Therapy for Nursing Students" to study the effectiveness of using programed instruction in a school of nursing. The study was conducted at the University of Rochester, and it was found that students who used the program obtained higher scores than those taught by traditional lecture methods; also there was a significant saving of time.§

A number of others have prepared programed instructional materials for teaching arithmetic for nursing.¶ ‖ Sacheim prepared "A Programmed Approach to the Circulatory System."**

* David J. Klaus. "The Art of Auto-Instructional Programming," *Audio-Visual Communications Review*, March-April 1961.

† Marie M. Seedor. *Introduction to Asepsis: A Programmed Unit in Fundamentals of Nursing*, Teachers College, Columbia University, Nursing Education Monograph No. 3, 1963.

‡ Marie M. Seedor. *Programmed Instruction for Nursing in the Community College*, Teachers College, Columbia University, 1963.

§ Josephine K. Crayton and J. P. Lysaught. "An Experiment with Programmed Instruction in Nursing Education," *NSPI J.* (Nat. Soc. for Programmed Instruction), 3:5, (May) 1964.

¶ Mabel Weaver and Vera J. Koehler. *Programmed Mathematics of Drugs and Solutions*, J.B. Lippincott Company, Philadelphia, 1964.

‖ George Sacheim and Robert Lewis. *Programmed Mathematics for Nurses*, The C.V. Mosby Company, St. Louis, 1964.

* * George Sacheim. *A Programmed Approach to the Circulatory System*, Stipes Publishing Company, Champaign, Ill., 1959.

New autoinstructional materials have been developed on obstetric and gynecologic disorders, cardiovascular diseases, diabetes, and diuretic agents for the Eli Lilly Company. This work was carried out at the American Institutes for Research. Some additional programs are listed in the bibliography.

From the above descriptions it is easy to see that a great deal has been done and is currently under way to develop autoinstructional materials for use in schools of nursing. This should do a great deal to individualize instruction and perhaps to shorten the time needed to cover course materials required to learn nursing skills.

STUDENT ACTIVITIES
IN THE LEARNING SITUATION

In the foregoing section discussion centered around aspects of teaching in the learning situation. Teachers, teaching methods, and teaching tools are vital factors in creating the climate conducive to learning. The quality of instruction can do much to improve opportunities for learning. However, the student must also make certain contributions to the learning situation if she is to benefit from the experience. The following chart indicates the nature of the interaction that should take place if opportunities for learning are to be optimal.

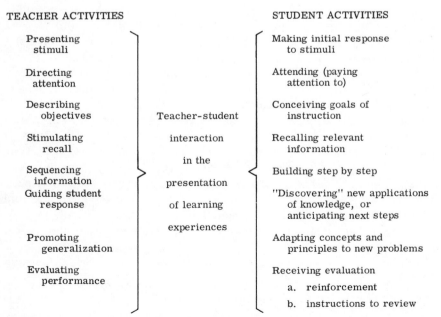

Figure 1 Teacher-student interaction in presenting the learning experience.

The nursing student's contributions to the learning situation include factors of interest, attitude, aptitude, and motivation. These all play important roles in the student's success in any educational program. To some extent, it is possible for instructors to direct student thinking and to develop student values in a way that will make learning experiences worthwhile. However, without the cooperation of the student, much if not most of the benefits of instruction can be lost.

It is the responsibility of the instructor to present the complete picture to the student and to introduce the knowledges, skills, and attitudes to acquaint the student with her ultimate responsibilities as a nurse. It is the responsibility of the student to recognize that the whole burden of education does not rest with the instructor. The student must participate as an active partner in this continuing, cooperative, on-going process.

In the charts which appear on pages 73 through 79, the authors have attempted to present graphically the steps involved in the preparation for and presentation of a learning experience by an instructor and its reception by the student. The activities on the part of the instructor and the student are illustrated in general terms in this example; however, it should help to clarify the kinds of interaction important to the instructional situation and to identify activities in terms of desired outcomes. Note that the plans include use of films and other audiovisual aids, field trips, lectures, and other teaching supplements as integral parts of the unit plan.

In nursing education it is important to recognize that there two types of learning experiences: one emphasizing technical knowledges and skills; the other involving learning experiences that will enhance and increase professional attitudes and values. The behaviors the student demonstrates in the acquisition of knowledges and skills have been identified by Bloom as the behaviors in the "cognitive domain,"* whereas development of appropriate sets of attitudes, appreciation, and values are considered to constitute behaviors in the noncognitive or "affective domain."†

Often in the stress and pressure of trying to achieve the objectives of the curriculum involving the academic, technical, and skills areas of the educational program, there may be tendencies to bypass opportunities to develop and encourage behaviors in the "affective domain." Attitudes, appreciation, and values cannot be taught in the same systematic way that we teach knowledges and skills. Education involving curriculum and course content has been explored to a far greater extent, and experience in this area is considerably greater. However, it would appear

* Benjamin S. Bloom. "Testing Cognitive Ability and Achievement," a chapter in *Handbook of Research on Teaching*, Nathan L. Gage (ed.), Rand McNally & Company, Chicago, 1963.

†D. R. Krathwohl, B. S. Bloom, and B. B. Masia. *Taxonomy of Educational Objectives: The Classification of Educational Goals, Handbook II: Affective Domain*, David McKay Company, Inc., New York, 1964, pp. 76-91.

Unit:

Objective:

OBJECTIVES (stated in behavioral terms)	CONTENT	(RELATED) LEARNING EXPERIENCES	TEACHER ACTIVITY	STUDENT ACTIVITY

E V A L U A T I O N

TEACHER EVALUATION

Review and re-evaluate the unit
in relation to student performance

1. Student objectives - based on changes in behavior
2. Content of unit
3. Associated (related) learning experiences
4. Teacher activity
5. Student activity

STUDENT EVALUATION

1. Written tests
2. Critical factor performance tests
3. Direct observation of critical incidents in daily performance on the ward
4. Standardized achievement tests
5. Class performance
6. Written assignments outside school

Figure 2 Schematic of activities involved in presenting a unit of instruction.

UNIT   Principles of nursing care of the patient who has had a personality change as a result of brain damage

UNIT OBJECTIVE   To assist the patient who has had a personality change to accept and adjust to his health condition utilizing the problem-solving technique

Objectives (Stated in Behavioral Terms)	Content	(Related) Learning Experiences	Teacher Activity	Student Activity

To know the vocabulary and definitions common in diseased conditions
To identify the common conditions causing personality change
To identify the special nerves and group of nerves affected
	Recognizing personality change as a physiological response of the body to a diseased condition
	A. Cause of problems
	  1. Obstruction, infection, hemorrhage
	    a. Subdural and epidural hematoma
	      1) Definition
	      2) Pathology
	    b. Brain trauma
	      1) Contusion
	      2) Concussion
	        a) Definition
	        b) Pathology
	    c. Brain tumors
	      1) Benign
	      2) Malignant
	    d. Cerebral arteriosclerosis
	      1) Definition
	      2) Pathology
		Viewing film	Distribute bibliography
			Distribute and orient student to Conference Guide
			
			Guide film discussion
				Draw head and its contents:
				1. Identify circulatory flow
				2. Identify nerves
				3. Locate vital centers
				4. Indicate areas of pathology in color
				Discussion of film

To contrast results of diagnostic tests with norms		Reading and reviewing the chart on diagnostic tests	Guide student in the discussion	Review of diagnostic findings
		Teaching rounds on selected patients with personality changes	Explain how each pathological condition causes problems in a patient Guide student in the discussion	Compare problems and personality changes observed on the patient during rounds Utilize Conference Guide in the discussion
To identify the signs and symptoms associated with the loss of sensory and motor function	B. Signs and symptoms presented by patient	Patient-centered conference on a patient who is having personality change as a result of a physiological condition	Guide discussion	Discuss nursing care necessary

(Continued)

Objective	Content	(Related) Learning Experiences	Teacher Activity	Student Activity
To construct a nursing care plan consistent with the medical care plan	C. Applied nursing care 1. Physiological		Assign student to an acutely ill patient who is having a change in personality (Cause of patient's problem based on content)	Evaluate why patient has a personality change due to a disease condition
To maintain a patent airway To demonstrate proper method of moving, turning, and lifting patient	a. Maintain oxygen supply b. Maintain body alignment c. Maintain function of regulatory mechanisms		Guide student in discussion	Preconference - before giving care Evaluates patient's problems

To check and record vital signs frequently and identify how they relate to increased intra-cranial pressure
To utilize the scientific principles involved in the care of the patient receiving hy-pothermia
	1) Vital signs
	2) Signs of increased intracranial pressure
	3) Hypothermia
	  a) Types
	    (1) Water mattress
	    (2) Mechanical
	    (3) Other
			Demonstrate and explain care of patient receiving hypothermia	Formulate a comprehensive care plan
				1. Place on Kardex

To identify the need for proper nutrition, body fluids, and elimination To know and utilize appropriate safety measures and protection necessary for the irresponsible patient	d. Maintain fluid and electrolytic balance e. Maintain elimination f. Maintain nutrition		Demonstration and preparation for intravenous infusion	Give care to assigned patient utilizing care plan Postconference - aftercare

(Continued)

Objective	Content	(Related) Learning Experiences	Teacher Activity	Student Activity
To determine and record levels of consciousness	2. Psychological a. Evaluating levels of consciousness	Patient-centered conference on a patient having emotional problems (based on content)	Orientation and preparation for - 1. Nursing rounds 2. Direct patient observation 3. Patient charts Guide student in discussion	Discussion conference after: 1. Nursing rounds 2. Reviewing charts
To recognize the signs of threat to emotional security	b. Negative vs. positive reactions			
To compare the relationship of emotional with organic illness	c. Interrelatedness of emotion and organic illness	Visit to a guidance clinic		Discussion conference after clinic visit
	d. Spiritual guidance available			
To develop a listening approach to allay patient fears			Assign student to a patient having an emotional problem (based on content)	Decide course of action and prepare a comprehensive care plan
To identify the social problems of a patient with personality change	3. Sociological a. Accepting goals in relation to limitations	Patient-centered conference on preparation of a patient for discharge Emphasize rehabilitative aspects	Present Guide for process recording Review charts of several patients Review Kardex and nursing care plans of several patients	Process recording on a selected patient utilizing Guide
To instruct the patient and the family in self care, adjustment to daily living, and community resources available	b. Community resources c. The patient's family	Resource persons - social worker and dietitian		Develop a home care plan as a guide for patient and family
To identify changes in personality that occur as a result of exogenous factors	Recognizing personality change as a physiological response of the body to toxic reactions			
To differentiate between physiological and psychological needs	A. Cause of problem - exogenous factors			

(Continued)

Objective	Content	(Related) Learning Experiences	Teacher Activity	Student Activity

To know the basic scientific principles that relate to the effect of alcohol on physiological changes	1. Drugs
	a. Bromides
	b. Alcohol
	  1) Chemical nature
	  2) Chemical reaction
	  3) Progressive pattern of alcohol addiction
		Viewing films
		"For Those Who Drink"
		"To Your Health"
			Guide film discussion	Review and react to film

To identify the signs and symptoms of progressive patterns of alcohol addiction				

To listen as patient expresses his needs and respond with sincerity and understanding	a) Signs and symptoms
	b) Phases
	  (1) Prodromal
	  (2) Basic
	  (3) Chronic			

To record fears, apprehensions, and verbalizations of patient				

To identify the social forces that are influencing factors in alcohol addiction	4) Cultural aspects of drinking
	a) Drinking patterns
	  (1) Nationality and ethnic groups
	  (2) Social drinking
	  (3) Attitudes
		Panel discussion
		Panel moderator from Department of Mental Hygiene - Rehabilitation Division
			Assign student to a patient with acute (or chronic) alcoholism (based on content)	Formulate nursing care plan
				Emphasis on covert problems

To identify alcoholism as a public health problem	5) Treatment a) Medical b) Psychotherapy			
To create an atmosphere conducive to establishing patient rapport in order to reinforce medical care plan				

(Continued)

Objective	Content	(Related) Learning Experiences	Teacher Activity	Student Activity
To know the community resources that are an aid in solving problems of the alcoholic To maintain composure in stress situations To converse with, instruct, and guide the family in adjusting to alcoholism as a disease	c) Community agencies 1-Alcoholics Anonymous and related groups	Visit to an AA meeting Patient-centered conference on an alcoholic patient with nutritional deficiencies	Make arrangements for students to attend an AA meeting Review Orientation Guide preparatory to meeting	Attend an AA meeting Conference following the meeting 1. Note and evaluate 12 steps to recovery 2. Report on talk with individual AA members 3. Evaluate their feelings about the program 4. Evaluate their progress 5. Report on talk with members of the family of an AA member 6. Review literature

(Continued)

TEACHER EVALUATION *

Review and re-evaluate the unit in relation to student performance:

1. Student objectives - based on behavior

2. Content of unit

3. Related learning experiences

4. Teacher activity

5. Student activity

The various tools the teacher may utilize to evaluate student progress in the various areas listed above are:

1. Written tests
   Essay
   Completion
   Situation
   Multiple choice
   Forced choice

2. Critical factor performance tests**
   (Scored using observational check list)

3. Direct observation of critical incidents in daily performance

4. Standardized achievement tests

This approach may be used in teaching fundamental nursing skills as well as in teaching various aspects of patient-centered care.

*See page 89
**See page 121

that many of the same principles that have been used successfully in achieving the changes of behavior in the cognitive domain could also prove useful in the development of behaviors in the affective domain. This approach may not prove to be the absolute answer but nevertheless could provide more emphasis than is presently given to the development of attitudes and values.

Krathwohl, Bloom, and Masia have formulated a general taxonomy of educational objectives in the affective domain to complement those previously developed for the cognitive domain.* The five levels of objectives in this hierachy are identified as:

Receiving (attending)—an awareness and willingness to receive
Responding—acquiescence, willingness, and satisfaction in response
Valuing—conscious control in the form of interest and attitudes
Organization—conceptualization and organization of a value system
Characterization by value or value complex—acting in accordance with
    internalized values

Just as in the cognitive domain, the highest levels of objectives are more difficult to attain. However, each learning experience may be viewed as an opportunity to help the student attend and respond to the values inherent in the nurse's role. Careful curriculum planning and implementation should help to achieve at least the lower levels of the objectives identified by Bloom and his associates.† It is conceivable that, as a result of attending and responding to planned learning experiences in which attitudes, appreciation, and responsibilities are stressed, the student may be capable of developing an integrated personal system of values to guide her to continue and pursue a career in nursing. The cultivation of a desirable set of values can do much to enhance the worth of an individual to herself, to her profession, and to society.

Bibliography

Abdellah, Faye G. "Methods of Identifying Covert Aspects of Nursing Procedures," *Nursing Research*, 6:4, (June) 1947.
Abdellah, Faye G., Beland, Irene L., Martin, Almeda, and Matheney, Ruth V. *Patient-Centered Approaches to Nursing*, The Macmillan Company, New York, 1961.
Bermosk, Loretta Sue, and Mordan, Mary Jane. *Interviewing in Nursing*, The Macmillan Company, New York, 1964.
Bloom, Benjamin S. *Taxonomy of Educational Objectives. Handbook I: Cognitive Domain*. Longmans, Green and Co., New York, 1956.

---

* Krathwohl *et al., loc. cit.*
† Benjamin S. Bloom. *Taxonomy of Educational Objectives. Handbook I: Cognitive Domain*. Longmans, Green and Co., New York, 1956.

Brown, Amy Frances. *Curriculum Development*, W.B. Saunders Company, Philadelphia, 1961.

Brown, Esther L. *Nursing for the Future*, Russell Sage Foundation, New York, 1948.

Crayton, Josephine K., and Lysaught, J. P. "An Experiment with Programmed Instruction in Nursing Education," *NSPI Journal* (National Society for Programmed Instruction), **3**:5, (May) 1964.

Dressel, Paul L., and associates. *Evaluation in Higher Education*, Houghton Mifflin Company, Boston, 1961.

Flanagan, John C. *et al*. *The American High School Student*, Houghton Mifflin Company, Boston, in press, 1966.

Gage, Nathan L. (ed.). *Handbook of Research on Teaching*, chapter by Benjamin S. Bloom on "Testing Cognitive Ability and Achievement," Rand McNally & Company, Chicago, 1963.

Gardner, John W. *Excellence*, Harper & Brothers, New York, 1961.

Klaus, David J. *The Art of Programmed Instruction*, American Institutes for Research, Pittsburgh, 1961.

Klaus, David J. "The Art of Auto-Instructional Programming," *Audio-Visual Communications Review*, March-April, 1961.

Krathwohl, D. R., Bloom, B. S., and Masia, B. B. *Taxonomy of Educational Objectives: The Classification of Educational Goals, Handbook II: Affective Domain*, David McKay Company, Inc., New York, 1964.

Maier, Norman R. F. *Principles of Human Relations*, John Wiley & Sons, Inc., New York, 1952.

Miller, Robert B. *A Suggested Guide to Functional Characteristics of Training and Training Equipment*, Technical Memorandum ML-TM-56-14, Maintenance Laboratory, Air Force Personnel and Training Research Center, Air Research and Development Command, Lowry Air Force Base, Colorado, May, 1956.

National League for Nursing. *Toward Excellence in Nursing Education*, The League, New York, 1964.

Sacheim, George. *A Programmed Approach to the Circulatory System*, Stipes Publishing Company, Champaign, Ill., 1959.

Sacheim, George, and Lewis, Robert. *Programmed Mathematics for Nurses*, The C.V. Mosby Company, St. Louis, 1964.

Sand, Ole. *Curriculum Study in Basic Nursing Education*, G. P. Putnam's Sons, New York, 1955.

Sand, Ole, and Belcher, Helen. *An Experience in Basic Nursing Education*, G.P. Putnam's Sons, New York, 1958.

Seedor, Marie M. *Introduction to Asepsis: A Programmed Unit in Fundamentals of Nursing*, Teachers College, Columbia University. Nursing Education Monograph No. 3, 1963.

Seedor, Marie M. *Programmed Instruction for Nursing in the Community College*, Teachers College, Columbia University, 1963.

Siegel, Laurence. *Contemporary Theories of Instruction*, Chapter 3 by Robert M. Gagné, "Instruction and the Conditions of Learning," Chandler Publishing Company, San Francisco, 1965.

Weaver, Mabel, and Koehler, Vera J. *Programmed Mathematics of Drugs and Solutions*, J.B. Lippincott Company, Philadelphia, 1964.

Selected References

Abdellah, Faye G. "Methods of Determining Covert Aspects of Nursing Problems as a Basis for Improved Clinical Teaching," unpublished doctoral dissertation Teachers College, Columbia University, 1955.

Abdellah, Faye G., and Levine, E. *Patients and Personnel Speak*: A *Method of Studying Patient Care*, U.S. Government Printing Office, Washington, D.C., U.S.P.H.S. Publication No. 527, 1957.

Anderson, Maja C. *Basic Patient Care*: A *Programed Introduction to Nursing Fundamentals*, W.B. Saunders Company, Philadelphia, 1965.

Aydelatte, Myrtle K. "The Use of Patient Welfare as a Criterion Measure," *Nursing Research*, 11:10-14, (Jan.) 1962.

Carter, Frances M. "The Critical Incident Technique in the Identification of the Patients' Perception of Therapeutic Patient-Patient Interaction on a Psychiatric Ward," *Nursing Research*, 8:207-12, 1959.

Corbally, J. E., Jr. "The Critical Incident Technique in Educational Research," *Educational Research Bulletin*, 35:57-62, 1956.

Covey, F., and Covey, E. "Improving the Hospital School of Nursing," Georgia State College of Business Administration, Atlanta, 1957.

Diedrich, P. B. *The Critical Incident Technique Applied to Medical Education*, Educational Testing Service, Princeton, Research Memo 54-9, 1954.

Gagné, R. M., and Bolles, R. C. "A Review of Factors in Learning Efficiency," chapter in *Automated Teaching: The State of the Art*, E. Galanter (ed.), John Wiley & Sons, Inc., New York, 1959.

Glickman, A. S., and Vallance, T. R. "Curriculum Assessment with Critical Incidents," *J. Applied Psychol.*, 47:329-35, 1958.

Goldfarb, A. "Use of the Critical Incident Technique to Establish Areas of Change Accompanying Psychotherapy: II. Relationship to Diagnostic Group," unpublished master's thesis, University of Pittsburgh, 1952.

Hahn, C. P. *Measurement of Individual Differences with Respect to Critical Job Requirements*, U.S. Air Force School of Aviation Medicine, San Antonio, Report No. 2. Project No. 21-29-014, 1954, (AIR-A24-54-FR).

Hart, Luna K. *The Arithmetic of Dosage and Solutions*: A *Programmed Presentation*, The C.V. Mosby Company, St. Louis, 1965.

Heidgerken, Loretta E. "Curriculum Study of Nursing at the Graduate Level," *Nursing Research*, 7:90, (June) 1958.

Hendershot, C. H. *Programmed Learning*: A *Bibliography of Programs and Presentation Devices*, Author, Bay City, Mich., 1964.

Jacques, Marceline E. *Critical Counseling Behavior in Rehabilitation Settings*, State University of Iowa, 1959.

Klaus, David J. "Programming the Impossible," paper presented at the first annual meeting of the National Society for Programmed Instruction, San Antonio, March, 1963.

Klaus, David J. "Strategies for the Automation of Instruction," paper presented at the Second Annual Meeting of the National Society for Programmed Instruction, San Antonio, April, 1964.

Krumboltz, John D. *Learning and the Educational Process*, Chapter I by Robert M. Gagné, "Educational Objectives and Human Performance," Rand McNally & Company, Chicago, 1965.

Massoth, Sister Mary Colletta, R.S.M. "Problems Encountered by Second-Year Students in Their Nursing Learning Experiences in a Selected School of Nursing," unpublished master's thesis, Catholic University of America, 1956.

Mellett, T. P. "The Use of the Critical Incident Technique to Establish Areas of Change Accompanying Psychotherapy: III. Differences Among Therapists," unpublished master's thesis, University of Pittsburgh, 1952.

Speth, E. W. "The Use of the Critical Incident Technique to Establish Areas of Change Accompanying Psychotherapy: I. Function of Age and Education," unpublished master's thesis, University of Pittsburgh, 1952.

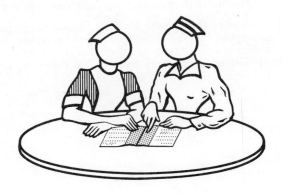

Critical Incident

Miss Midway, an intermediate student, had an evaluation conference with the clinical instructor. Later Miss Midway was observed rechecking the Expected Behavior Sheets she had received at the beginning of the course in psychiatric nursing. She was doing a self-evaluation using the Clinical Experience Record.

This is an effective critical incident for a student who was making an effort to evaluate her own performance in terms of the objectives of the course. She was checking her own behaviors against those listed as criteria for the course.

Chapter 6

Evaluation in

Terms of

Objectives

Evaluation in education is described in the *Encyclopedia of Educational Research* as a procedure which involves—

> . . . describing something, in terms of selected attributes, and judging the degree of acceptability or suitability of that which has been described. The "something" . . . may be any aspect of the educational scene, but it is typically (a) a total school program, (b) a curricular procedure, or (c) an individual or a group of individuals.*

Measurement is implicit in evaluation, but there is a distinction. Heidgerken describes measurement as an—

> . . . appraisal in terms of some fixed and absolute standard, whereas evaluation . . . implies the use of relative and flexible standards.†

Micheels and Karnes support this point of view:

> *Measurement* implies a precise, quantitative value which can be placed on a physical property or an outcome of instruction (a board is so many inches long or a student receives so many points on a particular test). *Evaluation* . . . is more comprehensive in nature and includes values which result from the exercise of judgment and more subjective appraisals (as well as from the use of strictly objective techniques).‡

Effective evaluation involves an assignment of values to the kinds of changes the student can demonstrate as a result of certain learning experi-

---

* Chester W. Harris (ed.). *Encyclopedia of Educational Research*, The Macmillan Company, New York, 1960, p. 482.
† Loretta E. Heidgerken. *Teaching in Schools of Nursing*, 3d ed., J.B. Lippincott Company, Philadelphia, 1965, p. 629.
‡ William J. Micheels and M. Ray Karnes. *Measuring Educational Achievement*, McGraw-Hill Series in Education, New York, 1950, p. 22.

ences. Evaluation should be based on course objectives in terms of new knowledges and skills the student has acquired. In this and succeeding chapters a number of questions about evaluation will be discussed.

1. Why is evaluation important?
2. What is to be evaluated?
3. What tools can we use?
4. How can we interpret the results?

WHY IS EVALUATION IMPORTANT?

One purpose of evaluation is to determine what the student has learned. In this sense "learning" implies more than mere rote memory or the comprehension of theoretical information. It implies capability to put theory into practice by actual application and demonstration. To approach the problem it is necessary first to have some insight and information about the student's state of knowledge before she entered the course. The changes in behavior that have taken place from the beginning of a course can provide supporting information to both the student and the instructor. Performance should be considered in the light of established objectives described in behavioral terms.

Changes in behavior can be measured in a variety of ways: through tests, by observation of performance, or on the basis of outcomes. Results of performance are usually reported in terms of scores on tests, grades assigned on the basis of some sliding scale of values, ratings, or rankings. Evaluation provides the student with information about the quality of performance. Thus, evaluation serves as feedback to help the student identify strengths and weaknesses.

Another important purpose of evaluation is to inform the instructor to what extent and how thoroughly materials and course content have been presented, and whether students have achieved the established objectives. Student achievement is heavily dependent on the nature and quality of instruction. This is true regardless of what teaching method is used. Consequently, evaluation serves to identify problems in teaching and teaching methods.

Evaluation also serves other purposes. It helps to identify strengths and weaknesses in educational objectives and in the curriculum. For example, if the students in School of Nursing A consistently achieve higher scores on licensing examinations and are more successful in careers as nurses than students from School B, it becomes rather obvious that the objectives of School B should be reviewed and re-examined. If the students taught by means of one approach to fundamentals of nursing consistently perform with a greater degree of effectiveness than students taught through another method, it should be obvious that the second method of teaching should be re-examined to determine where weaknesses exist and why these students fall short in comparison to others.

In addition, evaluation serves to motivate teachers and students alike. When teachers can identify and define weaknesses and strengths in the curriculum and in teaching methods, they have a better basis for overcoming problems and improving teaching. Evaluation can lead to systematic revision of curriculum and course content. When tests reflect achievement of course objectives, they provide a sound basis for evaluation. This is true of all types of tests, especially in critical factor performance tests where situations are built around specific objectives in terms of demonstrated performance. Information about strengths and weaknesses in performing nursing functions can provide the student with a better basis on which to plan for improvement. The student is often more inclined to try to improve her behavior when she knows where to start.

These are the purposes of evaluation: (1) identification of strengths and weaknesses in the objectives of an educational program; (2) identification of areas to be improved in the curriculum and in course content; (3) identification of weaknesses that may exist in the quality, the process, and the product of teaching; (4) identification of weaknesses and strengths in student performance; and (5) establishment of a basis for motivating both teachers and students toward improvement.

Boykin* and others (Rines,† Heidgerken,‡) describe a number of principles for effective evaluation. The present authors have grouped these in relation to objectives at three levels in an educational program: the school, the teacher, and the student.

Meeting School Objectives

1. *Evaluation should involve clear-cut concepts of the aims and needs of society, education, the school, and the individual.* Objectives for the over-all educational program must be periodically evaluated through qualitative and quantitative measures. To what extent are the objectives of the school being met? What degree of success are the graduates of this school achieving? How many actually go into nursing? How many leave the profession after a year or two? How many pursue advanced education and assume positions of increasing responsibility?

If follow-up studies reveal that the graduates of a particular school remain active practitioners in the profession and achieve more than a moderate degree of success in careers as nurses, it can be assumed that the school has been relatively successful in achieving its objectives. Evaluation in-

---

* L. L. Boykin. "What Is Evaluation?" *J. Educational Research*, **51**:531-33, 1958.
† Alice R. Rines. *Evaluating Student Progress in Learning the Practice of Nursing*, Teachers College, Columbia University, 1963, pp. 18-21.
‡ Heidgerken, *op. cit.*

dicates that the school is (1) adequately meeting the needs of society by providing competent nurses, (2) meeting the needs of education by providing effective teachers and teaching methods and the kind of climate conducive to learning, and (3) meeting the needs of the individual student by providing opportunities to acquire the kind of education and learning experiences that can lead to a career offering possibilities for self-realization, self-fulfillment, and self-direction.

2. *Evaluation should be a continuing, cooperative process.* Any educational institution is heavily dependent upon the interaction of administrators, faculty, and students. Responsibility for initiating changes in policy and organizational structure rests with the administrative body, who should work in close cooperation with the teaching staff. The establishment of objectives should be a cooperative endeavor. Policies and practices should be subject to periodic re-examination and review by the committee on objectives and by the faculty. No drastic changes should be made without complete orientation of the faculty as to the nature of the changes and the reasons for introducing them. The faculty should have an opportunity to voice their opinions about the feasibility of making changes and to consider the best methods for implementing the new ideas. (See Chapter 3.)

Often in a school of nursing some of the faculty are members of the "old guard." They resist all change and want teaching to remain "just the way we've always done it." Others have kept abreast of the rapid changes in the field of education and nursing and favor introducing some of the better innovations as part of the teaching program. This is bound to result in conflict. Every effort should be made to resolve such differences by an objective review of the policies and practices of the school. The basic purpose of this re-evaluation should be to identify strengths and weaknesses. In this way it should be possible to work constructively toward the establishment of sounder policies and to revise objectives in accordance with the needs of society, the school, and the student.

3. *Self-evaluation should take place periodically.* Self-evaluation at the school level should be a continuing, on-going, cooperative effort on the part of everyone involved directly or indirectly in the educational program. Objectives should be reviewed and updated on a periodic, systematic basis.

Meeting Teacher Objectives

1. *Evaluation should be comprehensive in scope.* What is the importance of evaluation for the teacher? To be meaningful, evaluation should be comprehensive, covering the student performance not only for the benefit of the student, but in terms of the quality of teaching offered. Instructors should endeavor to use the most effective methods to review teaching practice to determine how adequately they are meeting student needs in relation to educational objectives. Curriculum and course content should be

re-evaluated to make certain they are sufficiently flexible to provide worth-while learning experiences for the students.

2. *Evaluation should involve an intensive study of the changes that oc-cur in student behavior.* Was the teaching adequate? The degree and nature of changes in student behavior must be constantly evaluated to determine whether they are (1) the kinds of changes that indicate learning has taken place; (2) changes that can contribute positively to the student's growth and development, to increasing her skills and knowledge in preparation for a career in nursing; (3) changes that are sufficient or just barely meeting the goals and objectives of the curriculum; (4) changes that can be rein-forced for student retention; or (5) undesirable changes that should be overcome and eliminated.

3. *Evaluation should provide opportunities to improve teaching.* If stu-dents fail to meet the objectives of a unit or a course, it may be well to re-evaluate teaching methods. There may be insufficient emphasis on some aspects of the program. Was too much presented too soon? Do students re-quire the use of more teaching materials? Visual aids, film strips, closed-circuit television, autoinstructional programs, and other teaching devices often help to supplement teaching and lead to improved student perform-ance. Evaluation of student achievement to identify needs for improvement in teaching should be an implicit part of any educational program.

4. *Evaluation should be a continuing, on-going process of cooperation between teacher and student.* It is possible to learn through teaching. Eval-uation can serve to enhance and improve human relations between the teacher and the student. Creating an atmosphere of mutual respect and cooperation through evaluation can provide the basis for improving both teaching and learning. The old-time stigma of the evaluative situation should be reduced or if possible eliminated. Permitting and encouraging student cooperation in evaluation can be a valuable learning experience for both student and teacher.

There should be no "day of reckoning"; evaluation should be a constant and continuing process. Students should not anticipate evaluation in fear—it should be a constructive feature of each day's learning situation.

5. *Evaluation should provide the basis for counseling and guidance.* Evaluation should be used to plan for student growth. Objective evaluation provides the basis for counseling activities. Guidance through evaluation does more than advise students "just where they stand" in a class. A care-ful review of the facts based on a record of performance can lead to a con-structive plan for improvement. Counseling today involves helping students to help themselves by providing meaningful information about progress and by encouraging student participation in planning for future activities.

6. *Self-evaluation should be a part of teaching practice.* Evaluation of student performance often reveals information that can be used as the basis for making revisions in course content or the curriculum. It can also pro-

vide valuable information regarding the success or adequacy of the teaching methods used. Frequent review of teaching methods should be a periodic and systematic part of the teaching program. There are so many innovations in the field of teaching that it is worthwhile to take the time to review them and put the best of them into practical use in schools of nursing.

Meeting Student Objectives

1. *Evaluation should be a cooperative, continuing process between the student and the instructor.* How often have you heard a student "blame" a teacher for a poor grade. This student assumes the teacher alone is responsible for the grade on her evaluation report. In a school of nursing, the teacher is responsible for gathering data on the basis of student performance in daily class work, written assignments, quizzes, laboratory demonstrations, and in observing the student in the clinical area. The student is responsible for demonstrating to the instructor performance of a quality that represents her best efforts to meet established standards. Evaluation should be a cooperative effort.

When an atmosphere of cooperation is established, the teacher feels free to discuss with the student any incidents of deviation from the accepted standard. The student should welcome this discussion as a basis for planning appropriate action to overcome difficulties. Conversely, the student should feel equally free to approach the teacher at any time, assuming that "evaluation day" is not just at the end of a quarter or semester, but that evaluation is a continuing, on-going process every day. If a student feels free to seek assistance when she first senses a problem, she may be able to overcome it early. On the other hand, if a permissive atmosphere does not exist, early problems can magnify and often defeat the student. She may lose contact. The gap in information tends to widen. The mastery of new concepts is usually contingent upon earlier learning and provides the prerequisite to later learning. The student should relate new information to what she has already learned and should recognize the continuity.

2. *Evaluation should serve as an indication of degree of accomplishment.* Any time one person performs and another assesses performance, the performer wants to know how well he has done. Evaluation should communicate the degree of accomplishment. This is especially important in a school of nursing, because the student wants to know more than mere scores on tests, she wants to know how well she performs as a nurse. In most student-teacher relationships, it is possible to evaluate only the theory the student has learned. Seldom is there the wonderful opportunity for the student to demonstrate learning by actual practice in real life situations. Good feedback to the student about her handling of patient problems can be an important part of each day. Periodic teacher-student conferences should be welcomed by the student as opportunities to learn how much has been accomplished and what more must be done.

The student also has an obligation to the teacher. If a student has failed in some aspect of patient care, she should feel free to ask for clarification if she does not fully understand why she failed. She should seek opportunities for review if this seems indicated. The teacher should not bear the entire burden of deciding when students are having problems. Students should feel sufficiently mature to seek help when they need it and to feel free to find it.

3. *Self-evaluation should be an implicit part of the education program.* Many values accrue from self-evaluation. If instruction involves an adequate presentation of objectives, the student should be able to evaluate her own progress in relation to those objectives. The ability to be critical in assessing one's own performance is a mark of maturity. Self-evaluation is especially important to the student nurse because as a practitioner she will be responsible for evaluating the adequacy of the care she gives to her patients. Early development of the ability to assess one's own contribution to a situation can result in an improved quality of nursing. Self-evaluation can lead to self-direction.

These are the reasons we evaluate: (1) to obtain estimates of the achievement of the objectives of the school; (2) to provide meaningful information to the teacher to assist students and improve teaching methods; (3) to provide information to the student for self-improvement, growth, and development, and the achievement of personal goals in a socially acceptable manner; and (4) to provide information based on student performance and teaching effectiveness that can lead to modifications and improvements in the methods and materials used. Evaluation must be a cooperative and continuous process at every level in the educational situation, subject to constant re-examination and feedback.

Figure 3 shows the flow of activity in an evaluation program in a school of nursing. Evaluation begins with the development of objectives, their definition, and clarification. Following this, there is the development of curriculum objectives and course content for which learning experiences are selected and organized. Based on the administration of the program to the students, student performance should be evaluated in terms of the course and curriculum objectives. Periodically, there should be a re-evaluation of objectives and performance at all levels based on the experience gained using the curriculums and courses in the school program. Evaluation, then, is a cyclic process in which everyone must participate and cooperatively work toward improvement of the educational program of the school.

Trafford P. Maher summarized the situation during the Workshops of the Council of Member Agencies of the Department of Diploma and Associate Degree Programs.* He stated that we all have an obligation in our

* National League for Nursing. *Evaluation—The Whys and the Ways*, The League, New York, 1965, pp. 12-13.

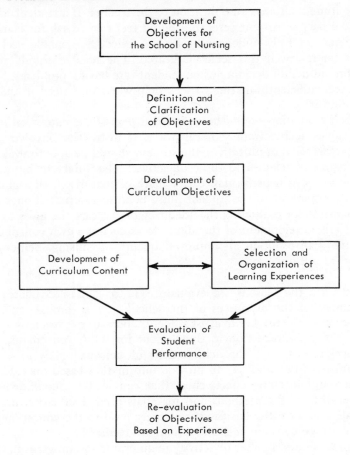

Figure 3   Graphic presentation of sequence in the development of objectives for a school of nursing.

commitments to evaluation, that: "For an evaluation to be maximally productive, it must be perceived as a deep personal educational experience for all involved." He emphasized that the reason we evaluate is to improve the total program and the effectiveness of the people in it from the standpoint of—

1. Values, loyalties, and commitments
2. Concepts of prevention (positive) and concepts of cure (negative)
3. Opportunities for satisfaction and service through nursing
4. Student growth and development
5. Personal and professional development

Bibliography

Boykin, L. L. "What Is Evaluation?" *J. Educational Research,* **51:**529-34, 1958.

Harris, Chester W. (ed.). *Encyclopedia of Educational Research,* The Macmillan Company, New York, 1960.

Heidgerken, Loretta E. *Teaching in Schools of Nursing,* 3d ed., J.B. Lippincott Company, Philadelphia, 1965.

Micheels, William J., and Karnes, M. Ray. *Measuring Educational Achievement,* McGraw-Hill Series in Education, New York, 1950.

National League for Nursing. *Evaluation—The Whys and Ways,* The League, New York, 1965.

Rines, Alice R. *Evaluating Student Progress in Learning the Practice of Nursing,* Teachers College, Columbia University, Monograph No. 5, 1963.

Selected References

Mayhew, Lewis B. "The Critical Incident Technique in Educational Evaluation," *J. Educational Research,* **49:**591-98, 1956.

Nelson, K. G., Bicknell, J. E., and Hedlund, P. A. *Development and Refinement of Measures of Teaching Effectiveness,* State Education Department, University of New York, 1956.

Shaycoft, Marion F., and Altman, J. W. *Procedure for Evaluation of Job Performance in Scientific Research,* American Institutes for Research, Pittsburgh, 1955 (AIR-A33-55-FR-109).

Shotwell, Anna M., Dingman, H. F., and Tarjan, G. "Need for Improved Criteria in Evaluating Job Performance of State Hospital Employees," *Am. J. Ment. Deficiency,* **65:**208-13, 1960.

Smith, E. R., and Tyler, Ralph W. "Appraising and Recording Student Progress," *Adventures in American Education,* Vol. III, Harper & Brothers, New York, 1942.

Sommermeyer, Lucille. "Applying the Critical Incident Technique to the Problem of Evaluating the Performance of Student Nurses in Nursing Situations," unpublished master's thesis, Boston University School of Nursing, 1954.

Tate, Barbara L. *Test of a Nursing Performance Evaluation Instrument,* National League for Nursing Research and Studies Service, New York, 1964.

Tschudin, Mary S., *et al. Evaluation in Basic Nursing Education,* G. P. Putnam's Sons, New York, 1958.

Weislogel, Mary H. *Procedures for Evaluating Research Personnel with a Performance Record of Critical Incidents,* American Institutes for Research, Pittsburgh, 1950 (AIR-A20-50-FR-16).

Wrightstone, J. Wayne, Justman, Joseph, and Robbins, Irving. *Evaluation in Modern Education,* American Book Company, New York, 1956.

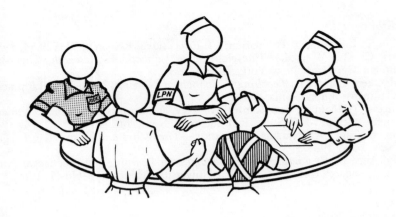

Critical Incident

Members of a curriculum committee were evaluating the course content in several areas during their annual curriculum evaluation meeting. A controversy arose over the definition and meaning of patient-centered nursing, total patient care, and comprehensive nursing.

Miss Farley, a medical-surgical nursing instructor stated, "We aren't talking the same language—What we need is a clarification of terms."

This is an effective critical incident on the part of the instructor in identifying and offering a solution to a problem. This is a constructive effort in dealing with co-workers.

Chapter 7

Evaluation in

Terms of

the Task

WHAT SHOULD WE EVALUATE?

The Task

The term "task" as it is used in this book refers to anything people do in connection with their work. In nursing a task could imply any kind of systematic behavior: comforting a patient, teaching home care, performing procedural functions such as irrigating a tracheostomy tube, or performing the complex task of identifying the covert problems an aged and depressed patient might have in facing surgery. In any profession or occupation there are many kinds of tasks, each of which requires a specific type of action or series of actions.

If we hope to evaluate a person's actions, we must approach the matter through a delineation of the tasks that person performs in the course of her daily activities. The behaviors manifested in performing each assignment provide the basis on which to evaluate the effectiveness or ineffectiveness of the outcomes. However, until we understand all aspects of the tasks to be performed, it would be difficult to ascertain whether the behaviors demonstrated were appropriate or inappropriate.

Evaluation of tasks in nursing, then, must take into consideration descriptions of each unit of the work a nurse must do, and this information must be broken down into units and described step by step to identify the kinds of behavior required to accomplish each phase of the work.

THE TASK ANALYSIS APPROACH

Breaking down an activity into components is a procedure known as task analysis. Gagné describes a task as the "smallest unit of performance which can be identified as having a distinct and independent purpose."* Any occupation, regardless of the work involved, can be subdivided into a series of small steps. When these are adequately performed in proper sequence, it should be possible to complete a unit of work in a satisfactory manner.

Teaching people to perform tasks is considerably easier if there are step-by-step descriptions to serve as guides to teaching and learning. The detailed statements about tasks are known as *task descriptions.* The most effective types of task descriptions include information about (1) the person (title or job level), (2) the equipment to be used, (3) the environment in which the work will be done, (4) the other people who may interact with the person or the equipment, and (5) anticipated outcomes. The more accurate the task description, the more useful it can be in guiding action.

For purposes of illustration we have chosen a very basic, well-known task, that of taking a patient's blood pressure. To those who have learned how to do this procedure, it now appears to be quite simple. However, to someone who has never used a manometer and who has never taken a patient's blood pressure, each of the steps defined here is quite new and important. Using these steps it should be possible within a short time to teach the student the procedure. Once she has seen and returned the demonstration, she should be able to use the task description to guide her practice of this task.

Several sample descriptions are given below. The important steps are discussed by referring to Activity 1 and Activity 2.

Performance Description—Taking Blood Pressure†

JOB TITLE: Nurse or appropriate member of health team
ACTIVITY 1: Takes patient's blood pressure.
OBJECT ACTED UPON: Patient's arm or leg (usually the left arm).
INFORMATION GUIDING ACTION: Recall, nursing or doctor's orders, nursing procedure book.
TOOLS: Pressure cuff, manometer, stethoscope, alcohol sponge.
ACTION: Executes a procedure.
1. Explains necessity for procedure and any unusual circumstances to the patient.
2. Sees that the patient is in a comfortable recumbent or sitting position, unless otherwise ordered. The recumbent position is preferred. However, in the diagnosis of certain types of hypertension,

---

* John D. Krumboltz. *Learning and the Educational Process*, Chapter I, "Educational Objectives and Human Performance," by Robert M. Gagné, Rand McNally & Company, Chicago, 1965.

† This performance description was prepared by Angeline Marchese Jacobs, R.N., in connection with a project on vocational education and the development of generalizable skills conducted by the American Institutes for Research for the Ford Foundation.

the blood pressure is taken in the standing position as well as in sitting and recumbent positions.

3. Position patient's arm so that it is supported at heart level. Usually the left arm is used. In repeated blood pressure measurements, the same arm should be used, for comparative purposes. When measurements are made on the leg, the cuff is placed above the knee and the stethoscope over the popliteal space (behind the knee). The manometer should be placed so that the nurse can achieve an eye-level view of the scale, to prevent parallax.

4. Removes patient's gown from arm.

5. Expels any air in the pressure cuff by squeezing it.

6. Wraps cuff (comfortably) around the arm above the elbow (so that the tubes from it will not be over the antecubital space, where the stethoscope will be placed).

7. Finds pulsation of the brachial artery (the inner aspect of the bend of the arm) by palpation.

8. Places the stethoscope in ears.

9. While palpating the radial pulse, inflates cuff until manometer indicates 10 to 30 mm of mercury beyond obliteration of the radial pulse. This prevents discomfort from unnecessary pressure of the cuff.

10. Places bell or diaphragm of stethoscope over brachial artery in antecubital space.

11. Releases air very slowly from cuff by using valve on inflation bulb, until the first audible sound is heard. This is the systolic pressure.

12. Notes (mentally) manometer reading at the systolic pressure.

13. Continues to release air until there is a complete cessation of sound.

14. Notes (mentally) the manometer reading at the last audible sound. This is the diastolic pressure.

15. Removes stethoscope from ears.

16. Releases cuff from patient's arm (or leg).

17. Records systolic and diastolic pressures along with patient's name on note pad (e.g., 120/80).

18. Wipes bell and ear pieces of stethoscope with alcohol sponge to prevent cross-contamination.

19. Transcribes blood pressure reading from note pad to patient's chart.

20. Reports excessively low or high pressure to nurse in charge or doctor. Excessively low pressure (below 80 systolic) may indicate severe blood loss or shock. Excessively high pressure may necessitate phlebotomy (surgical or dry) in some cases of severe hypertension.

COMPLETION INDICATOR: Blood pressure is properly recorded on patient's chart.

Detailed Analysis of Activity 1

1. *The task is identified.* Taking blood pressure.

2. *The object involved is described.* The patient's arm or his leg (a portion of the patient's body).

3. *The basis for initiating action is specified.*

a. Recall—if blood pressure is a routine part of admitting a patient to the hospital room, the action is initiated on the basis of recall of this general practice.

b. Nursing or doctor's orders—depending on the patient's condition, there may be need periodically to take blood pressure. This is indicated either in nurse's or doctor's orders.

c. Nursing procedure book—if the nurse is new and she is approaching her first patient, she may need to check the procedure in the nursing procedure book.

4. *Equipment is described (if equipment is involved).* Pressure cuff, manometer, stethoscope, alcohol sponge. These are the items needed to take blood pressure. The nurse should know this and should prepare all these items before she begins to take the patient's blood pressure.

5. *The action is described.* See steps 1 through 20 in the Activity Description. Each of these steps is important in taking blood pressure. The omission of one or several could result in an inaccurate reading.

6. *Final action or outcome is described.* In taking blood pressure the final action is to record the blood pressure on the patient's chart. When this is done, the action is completed. This *is* verifiable and can be checked if necessary by repeating the procedure.

The following is a more complex task.

Performance Description—Comforting Patient*

JOB TITLE: Nurse or appropriate member of health team.

ACTIVITY 2:   Comforts patient.

OBJECT ACTED UPON: Patient.

INFORMATION GUIDING ACTION: Recall, diagnosis, personal and family health history, socioeconomic background, signs and symptoms patient presents, medical care plan.

TOOLS: Knowledge of patient's problem.
    The chart—nurse's notes.
    Diagnostic tests.
    Knowledge of source and action of drugs

ACTION: Identifies cause of problem.
    Prepares a comprehensive care plan.

1. Listens to patient.
2. Provides assurance. (Is honest and realistic. Avoids platitudes.)
3. Reacts to patient's expressed needs.
4. Reassures patient that his choice of physician is a good one.

* This performance description was prepared by Angeline Marchese Jacobs, R.N., in connection with a project on vocational education and the development of generalizable skills conducted by the American Institutes for Research for the Ford Foundation.

5. Respects patient's privacy and opinion.
6. Holds information given patient in confidence.
7. Explains preparation for diagnostic tests and surgery in a manner and vocabulary the patient can understand.
8. Arranges for diversional therapy: i.e., TV, radio, mobile library.
9. Arranges for patient to talk with others on the ward who have positive results of surgery.
10. Provides for comfort and safety of the patient.
11. Arranges for visitation of clergyman, if indicated.

COMPLETION INDICATOR: Patient's anxiety is reduced.

REMARKS: Nurse's capability in this task, along with her general competence is probably—
1. Why she was attracted to the field of nursing.
2. Satisfying her need to be of service and the reason she remains in the field

Detailed Analysis of Activity 2

1. *The task is identified.* Comforting the patient.

2. *The object involved is described.* The patient. Here, no single part of the patient's body is involved—the patient himself is the object.

3. *The basis for initiating action is specified.*

a. Recall—The nurse from previous experience will know the signs and symptoms that indicate the need for providing comfort. She will recall learning experiences in comforting patients.

b. Expressed fear on the part of the patient. In some cases the patient will verbalize his fears. If he does, this is an indication that should initiate comforting action on the part of the nurse.

4. *Equipment is described* (if any equipment is involved). The tools in this activity are the nurse's knowledge, her ingenuity, and her judgment as well as her tact, patience, and understanding.

5. *The action is described.* The action in comforting a patient will vary depending on the kind and amount of assurance the patient needs. There is no easy scale or indicator which tells the nurse when the assurance has been sufficient. She must "sense" this from the reaction of the patient. In some instances the nurse provides the best comforting action by merely listening while the patient unburdens some of the thoughts that are troubling him.

6. *Final action or outcome is described.* Final action is not so easy to measure; the outcome is subtle. One indication of success will be that the patient is more relaxed; his fear and anxiety may be reduced. It is often difficult to tell the point at which this occurs. Relaxation may be one sign; a more optimistic attitude is another. The signs may be difficult to detect if the person is not expressive. However, it is usually not too difficult to tell if the heavy depression or fears persist, because the patient will not be relaxed and he may continue to verbalize his fears, in addition to showing

psychologic changes caused by prolonged stress such as lack of appetite, temperature elevation, or sighing. If this is the case, and further efforts and assurance fail, the student should seek assistance of the head nurse or the doctor, or possibly she should enlist the assistance of some member of the patient's family.

CONSIDERATIONS IN DEVELOPING PERFORMANCE DESCRIPTIONS

A performance description is intended as a list of sequential behaviors in terms of interaction of people, equipment, and the environment in which they perform. The success of this approach is contingent upon the accuracy and completeness of the information presented. Miller cautions that in developing descriptions several points should be considered:*

1. *Avoid inaccurate assumptions.* Often people tend to generalize and to make inaccurate assumptions on the basis of inadequate information. For example, at first glance someone observing a nurse taking blood pressure using the manometer may jump to the conclusion that because the nurse is required to read the manometer scale she should know mathematics. This is an inaccurate assumption. Mathematics is not needed to do this task, not even simple arithmetic. The nurse merely records what she reads on the scale. An accurate assumption would be that the nurse should know how to read scales.

2. *Avoid underestimating prerequisite skills.* In describing performance it is important to recognize the prerequisite skills needed. An inexperienced observer may tend to overlook important skills because their use may not be apparent. The very simple steps taken in combining reagents with the urine to test for sugar, albumin, or acetone require some understanding of the interaction of the substances being combined. Underestimating requirements can impair the efficiency of a description.

3. *Avoid emphasizing only normal conditions.* Normal conditions do not always prevail. Contigencies, emergencies, or unanticipated problems do happen, and these should be listed so that someone undertaking an activity for the first time will be aware of these possibilities. She should be told *what might happen* in the way of deviations from the usual situation and *what she should do* to cope with the unusual situation. Thus, when performance descriptions are developed, they should include contingencies and what to do about them.

4. *Avoid overemphasizing abnormal conditions.* Sometimes in an effort to include the unusual conditions, there may be a tendency to overcorrect and concentrate unduly on contingencies which rarely occur. For example,

* B. von Haller Gilmer (ed.). *Industrial Psychology*, chapter on "Problems Related to Work" by Robert B. Miller, McGraw-Hill Book Company, Inc., New York, 1961, pp. 373-80.

if a nurse is suctioning a tracheostomy tube she will need to know how to aspirate. If the tube should slip, the nurse should know how to adjust it, or even how to keep the opening patent if the tube is not reinsertable. However, she need not know how to perform a tracheostomy. If cardiac arrest occurs, the nurse should know how to give closed cardiac massage to meet the emergency; or if respiration fails, the nurse should be able to give mouth-to-mouth resuscitation, but she need not know how to do open heart surgery. When a postoperative patient becomes deeply depressed, the nurse should be able to cope with this emotional disturbance by reassuring the patient that the medication will soon take effect and that he will feel much better before long. To cope with these problems, the nurse need not be a clinical psychologist or a psychiatrist.

THE PURPOSES OF
PERFORMANCE DESCRIPTIONS

Performance descriptions serve many purposes.

1. *Selection Requirements*

Specifications of the aptitudes required for an activity are important to effective selection. For example, nurses must learn to read thermometers. One of the aptitudes involved is scale reading. Accurate performance descriptions would help nurse educators to identify this aptitude. Knowledge of important aptitudes required to perform nursing functions could lead to the development of aptitude tests for screening applicants for schools of nursing. It has been found that both time and funds can be saved if students are selected on the basis of aptitude for a particular kind of work.

2. *Job Design*

Detailed descriptions covering all aspects of a job can provide better insight into the step-by-step sequence required to do a job. Information of this type can lead to a reorganization of the steps, possibly the elimination of repetitive action, or the combination of several steps to improve performance. Good use of performance descriptions may lead to the combination of several tasks which can be carried on simultaneously by one person in situations where two or more people are used less efficiently.

3. *Equipment Design*

Performance descriptions can lead to improvements in the equipment used to do many kinds of work. A simple example is the use of the new type of resealable mastic on blood pressure cuffs. Heretofore it was necessary to either clip or hook the cuff around the patient's arm. Now, it is merely necessary to press the end of the wrapper against itself, and it will adhere without need for hooks or clips. Another example is the development of disposable syringes which need no longer be sterilized after they are used. They are designed for one-time use and disposal. Disposable enemas are still another innovation reducing and eliminating the need for tedious preparation and clean-up.

4. Teaching

Miller suggests that good performance descriptions can provide important information for teaching people to perform various kinds of work.* The identification of step intervals makes it possible to sequence the instruction in a logical manner so that the student will know the order in which the steps are to be taken.

5. Learning

Not only is the performance description a valuable aid to teaching, it can be equally useful to the student. Once preliminary instruction has been provided, a student can use the description to guide her in checking performance and to review each step involved. The student can check the description for purposes of refreshing the steps in a procedure learned sometime in the past.

6. Evaluation of Performance

A performance description in itself is not intended as an evaluation tool; however, the information can provide the basis on which to check performance for accuracy and step-by-step sequence. In this sense, the description can provide task criteria. The descriptions also make it fairly easy for instructors to develop tests of performance on small segments of work.

Task descriptions of the type presented help to provide the systematic breakdown of components of a task for job simplification in developing fundamental nursing skills.

What Is Skill?

Skill can be described as an organized pattern of proficiency in performing a task with a certain degree of speed, accuracy, and coordination. Smith† indicates that all actions involved in a task may not require skill; some are so simple and basic that almost anyone could do them. For example, almost anyone can apply a bandage or a dressing. However, it requires skill to change a colostomy dressing, because certain knowledges and dexterity are combined in performing this function.

* Robert M. Gagné. *Psychological Principles in System Development*, Chapter 6, "Task Description and Analysis," by Robert B. Miller, Holt, Rinehart and Winston; Inc., New York, 1962, p. 190.

† Robert G. Smith, Jr. *The Development of Training Objectives*, Research Bulletin 11, Human Resources Research Office, George Washington University, 1964, p. 56.

Inserting an airway is an example of a somewhat simple procedure that requires skill. In the chart on page 104 each of the component steps is identified, and the relationships of all the components to the task are shown as first- and second-level knowledges and skills. A nurse would not be able to recognize the symptoms and signs of an air passage obstruction unless she possessed some knowledge about the respiratory tract and the respiratory system. In order to know *how to relieve the obstruction*, she would need to know the causes of the obstruction, the procedures to relieve an obstruction, and the equipment needed. In order to obtain and maintain a patent airway, she must make periodic observations on the patient and check the adequacy of the equipment. The combination of the first-level knowledges and skills makes it possible for the nurse to insert an airway successfully.

Descriptions of tasks and the critical behaviors required to perform tasks imply the need for communicating information about the task and the behaviors in terms that will be readily understandable to everyone and that will mean the same to everyone. There is need for a glossary of nursing tasks and terms—a taxonomy. This need is discussed in the following section.

A TASK TAXONOMY
FOR NURSING FUNCTIONS

The use of task descriptions requires rather extensive knowledge not only of the task to be performed but of the terminology or language to describe each step in the procedure. Because of the growing need for accurate information for both teaching and learning purposes, it would be desirable for a group of nurse educators and practitioners to undertake the development of taxonomies for nursing: a classification of tasks in a hierarchy of importance and a glossary of technical nursing terms.

A task taxonomy would serve to establish the kinds of components or skills involved in each task and would present various levels of tasks in relation to one another, beginning with the simplest types of functions and moving toward the more complex procedures requiring combinations of knowledges and skills of first and second levels of difficulty.

The terms in a taxonomy of this type should be standardized so that the descriptions mean the same to everyone who uses the classification scheme. For this reason it would be desirable to develop a glossary of terms, not in the usual manner of glossaries, but by including and excluding terms on the basis of their relationship to each other. Miller proposed a glossary of this type as a means for clarifying communication between teacher and student in the presentation of a complex task.* He cited as an

---

* Gagné, *op. cit.*, p. 193.

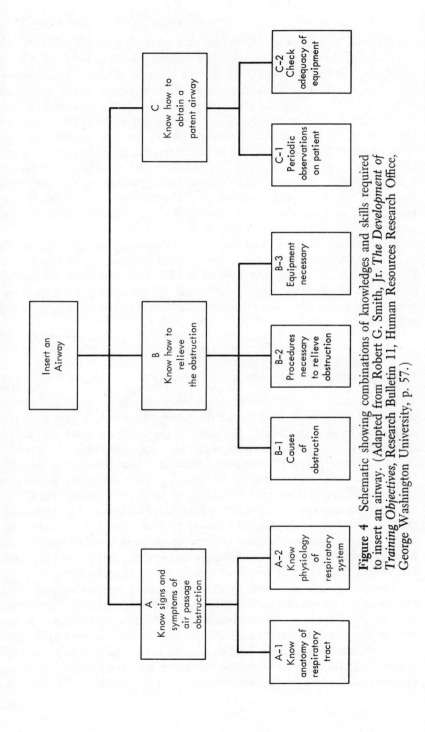

Figure 4 Schematic showing combinations of knowledges and skills required to insert an airway. (Adapted from Robert G. Smith, Jr. *The Development of Training Objectives*, Research Bulletin 11, Human Resources Research Office, George Washington University, p. 57.)

example the need to teach a student how to distinguish forms of life in a course in biology. The very general terms "animal life" and "plant life" are not sufficiently explicit to help the student to distinguish one from the other. However, if we use the terms "photosynthesis" and "carbon synthesis," we have an analytic and descriptive basis for differentiating one form of life from another.

A glossary of nursing terms that provided clarification and distinction of descriptions of the language of nursing would do a great deal to improve instructor-student communication. If terms were standardized, it would be possible to move to descriptions of tasks in a more systematic manner.

The development of a taxonomy of this type would be an important contribution to the field of nursing, particularly to nursing education.

Bibliography

Gagné Robert M. "Human Functions in Systems," *Psychological Principles in System Development*, Holt, Rinehart, and Winston, Inc., New York, 1962.

Krumboltz, John D. *Learning and the Educational Process*, Chapter I, "Educational Objectives and Human Performance," by Robert M. Gagné, Rand McNally & Company, Chicago, 1965.

Miller, Robert B. "Problems Related to Work," chapter in *Industrial Psychology*, B. von Haller Gilmer (ed.), McGraw-Hill Book Company, Inc., New York, 1961.

Miller, R. B. A *Method for Man-Machine Task Analysis*, Technical Report 53-137, Wright Air Dev. Center, Wright-Patterson Air Force Base, Ohio, 1953.

Miller, R. B. "Task Description and Analysis," chapter in *Psychological Principles in System Development*, Robert M. Gagné (ed.), Holt, Rinehart, and Winston, Inc., New York, 1962.

Miller, R. B., and Van Cott, H. P. *The Determination of Knowledge Content for Complex Man-Machine Jobs*, American Institutes for Research, Pittsburgh, 1955 (AIR-A93-55-FR-115).

Smith, Robert G., Jr. *The Development of Training Objectives*, Research Bulletin 11, Human Resources Research Office, George Washington University, 1964.

Critical Incident

At a meeting of the curriculum committee of faculty representatives from various areas in the nursing program, Mrs. Redman, the Director of Education, asked each member to review her teacher-made tests in relation to course content and curriculum objectives. Miss France, the faculty representative from maternal and child health, reviewed her test questions individually for the group and stated she had done an item analysis on the test and felt the objectives were being met since 95 per cent of her pupils had passed the test.

This is a critical incident. It is ineffective behavior on the part of Miss France. An item analysis would not necessarily indicate the school objectives were being met. In addition, the fact that 95 per cent of her pupils passed the test does not indicate that the course content was covered on the test. In either case, the questions may not have been relevant to the course objectives, and the students may have known the material from previous learning or were knowledgeable from emphasis placed on the material by the teacher but not listed in the course content. Appropriate behavior on Miss France's part would have been to relate each question to the specific area in the course content material and to the specific objectives to be covered.

Chapter 8
The Tools
of Evaluation

In preceding chapters the conditions of evaluation have been established: objectives, performance, and behavior are the bases for determining degrees of change.

Many methods have been devised for measuring the changes that take place as a result of learning. These include a wide variety of tests, some standardized on a national basis and available in printed form; others, teacher-made tests sampling the course content. In addition to the so-called tests of change there are other methods for evaluating changes in behavior based on direct observation of performance.

In this chapter we will discuss some of the many tools of evaluation, their advantages and limitations.

PAPER-AND-PENCIL TESTS, QUESTIONNAIRES, AND INTERVIEWS

Essay Examinations

One of the oldest forms of written tests is the essay examination. It has been the contention of many educators that essay examinations provide the best measure of the student's ability to organize information and to think in a creative manner. One advantage is that students must think of the answers when they write essays as contrasted with being given a series of answers from which they can make a choice on multiple-choice tests. Educators believe there is great advantage to stimulating and motivating students to think and write, and that the freedom of response tends to promote critical thinking and to elicit evidence of attitudes and values.

Allport defines the essay examination as:

> . . . a relatively free and extended written response to a problematic situation or situations (question or questions), which intentionally or unintentionally reveals information regarding the structure, dynamics, and functioning of the student's mental life as it has been modified by a particular set of learning experiences.*

He cites several distinctive features of essay examinations which endorse their use in cases where there is sufficient time and where objective short-answer tests do not provide enough information about the student: (1) The essay is useful for testing "higher-order" thinking and the intellectual outcomes of education. (2) The essay provides opportunities to make inferences concerning personal and social learning. (3) The essay provides information regarding the individual that can serve to guide future teaching. Unexpected insights are provided through responses to examination questions. This is not possible when multiple-choice tests are used; since the decision about responses is limited to those provided among the choices, no spontaneity is evident.

The critical factor in the use of essay examinations is in the construction of the questions to be used. Whereas the intent of objective test items is to elicit an exact response to a given question, the purpose of the essay question is to allow sufficient freedom to permit and encourage an extended response. Allport states that the more precise and exact the nature of the question, the less value it has in terms of testing free expression for projective purposes. Essay questions should pose problems which the student is required to solve in the sense of using knowledges and information from learning experiences to provide solutions, rather than applying the knowledge directly in the form of an exact answer to a precisely stated question. The best essay questions put the student into a new situation in which he is challenged to adapt and use the learning experiences being tested. The examinee is encouraged to use his own "frame of reference" in responding as opposed to having the frame of reference imposed upon him by the nature of the question and the given choices. Thus the essay tests judgment, the ability to organize one's thinking, and the ability to express ideas in an orderly and coherent fashion as compared with responses drawn almost entirely from memory.

The challenge to the instructor comes in the scoring of examinations using essay responses. Sims† suggests the following as guidelines to those who attempt to score essay examinations: (1) use an inductive method of evaluation; (2) distinguish data reflecting learning experiences from those

---

* George W. Allport. "The Use of Personal Documents in Psychological Science," *Social Science Research*, Monograph, No. 49:12, 1942.

† Verner M. Sims. "The Essay Examination Is a Projective Technique," *Educ. and Psychol. Measurement*, 8:15, (Jan.) 1948.

reflecting information about the personality of the student; (3) identify what is to be scored and develop a systematic method for making inferences from the data; (4) read the essays to determine what the student has learned, rather than merely summing up points; (5) beware of making too many generalizations based on single examples of essay responses.

In nursing education, there are numerous situations in which the use of essay examinations may be desirable. Much can be learned about attitudes, values, and appreciations the student has regarding specific learning experiences as expressed in essay form. This form of test should be especially useful in areas where attempts are being made to broaden the scope of student thinking or to change and modify basic attitudes regarding social problems, nursing care to patients in disadvantaged environments, or the care of elderly patients, or those who are mentally ill.

Short-Answer Tests

The most popular form of paper-and-pencil tests is the short-answer variety. There are a number of formats: multiple choice, true and false, comparison or matching of items, forced choice, free response, sentence completion, and filling in missing words. Short-answer tests can be useful measures of precisely the extent to which students have mastered theoretical and practical information presented in textbooks, lectures, demonstrations and laboratory experiments, and outside reading. They are not generally useful as measures of performance of motor skills unless such skills can be simulated through the use of pencil and paper.

Spaulding* developed a useful set of instructions for item writers who seek to construct short-answer tests for maximum effectiveness in ascertaining what the student has learned.

1. Select a task that is relevant and important with respect to the trait or ability to be measured, or one that involves behavior similar to that which it is desired to measure.
2. Define the task in clear-cut terms that are readily understood. This does not imply that the task cannot be complex. It does mean that there should be a clear description of the task as opposed to one that is buried in lengthy, wordy descriptions.
3. The formulation of the problem should not be more complex than the task requires. This applies not only to the language used to describe the problem, but also to the nature of the concepts needed to understand and solve it. Avoid the use of tricks or puzzles since these contribute little that is relevant to the task.
4. Analyze and evaluate the difficulty or complexity of all the problems. Emphasis should be placed on requiring the examinee to do a difficult task as opposed to requesting that he do the task in a difficult way.

* Geraldine Spaulding. "Memo on Item Writing," unpublished document prepared for the American Institutes for Research, Pittsburgh, 1950.

5. State the problem clearly, accurately, and completely in language that is readily understood. Make simple, direct, straightforward statements. Be sure of what you want to state as the problem and then state it in the way you mean it. Avoid lengthy, involved, or difficult sentence structure.

6. When the problem is complex, it is often preferable to use a separate sentence to ask the question, rather than attempt to incorporate both the statement of the problem and the question in one sentence.

7. Avoid negative statements as much as possible. A good test for the need for using the negative form is to ask yourself: (a) am I really interested in the student's ability to select the wrong answer; and (b) could this question be stated just as well in a positive way?

8. Use the same frame of reference for all choices. Independent choices should not require different interpretations of the stem.

9. If you want to measure judgment, understanding, reasoning, or the ability to perform a task, use a novel situation in the problem. In this way it is possible to test more than mere memory. Thus, it is desirable not to use questions directly from a textbook or workbook in a form the students may recognize and answer from memory.

10. Make an effort to include all or nearly all of the problem in the stem of an item. It should not be necessary to read all the choices in order to determine what the problem is about.

11. The student should not have to make inferences. The stem should be sufficiently clear and explicitly stated.

12. Avoid unnecessary descriptive materials. State the problem situation as precisely and accurately as possible.

13. If you plan to use incomplete sentences, test them by restating them in the form of a question. If it is not possible to make the conversion easily, apparently the problem has not been explicitly formulated.

14. Each of the choices should cover the same extent of information.

15. The stem of the item should not make untruthful implications about the choices. In other words, there should be no statement to the effect that all the choices are facts if they are not. Therefore, avoid using statements such as "Which of the following facts best describes the muscular system?" if all the statements are *not* facts.

16. Make the choices as brief as possible.

17. Do not use the choice "None of the above" unless there is just one strictly precise answer.

Spaulding* offers a checklist to help item writers determine how well the test meets the criteria described above. Test the test by asking yourself the following questions:

* Geraldine Spaulding, *loc. cit.*

1. Is the problem or question a useful one for the defined purposes of the test?
2. Have the conditions of the problem been clearly and accurately set forth in the stem of the item?
3. Does the examinee understand exactly what is to be done?
   a. Will he understand that he is to make a choice from those offered?
   b. Will he be able to decide what specifications the correct answer must fulfill?
4. Are the choices similar in all respects except the one crucial factor involved in the problem?
   a. Are they similar in grammatical structure?
   b. Are they approximately the same length?
   c. Are they similar in complexity, precision, and the amount of hedging or qualification involved?
   d. Are they similar with respect to the interpretation of the problem?
   e. Are wrong choices not too obvious by comparison with the correct choice?
5. Is the correct choice a precise, neat, correct answer to the problem, not only from the standpoint of information, but from the standpoint of grammar and thought?
6. Are the wrong choices clearly and definitely wrong without being subject to argument or qualification?
7. Is the selection of the right answer an accurate reflection of the basic problem in the item? Will this fact be clear to the examinee?

Engelhart* suggests the following as guidelines for the development of objective tests:

1. Distribute the items proportionately in relation to the emphasis and stress placed upon the content during the teaching of the materials.
2. Determine which materials can be tested most easily for application of principles, solution of novel problems, interpreting data, or the use of other kinds of skills.
3. Decide which materials lend themselves best to multiple-choice items and which would be tested better using other forms of items.
4. Prepare specific directions for each kind of item in the test.
5. If an answer sheet is to be used, give an illustration of an item with the correct answer designated in the format of the answer sheet.
6. If maps, charts, or illustrations are used, make certain that the stem and choices of the items use letters or numbers that correspond with the designations on the illustrative materials.
7. Prepare a key and have someone check it for accuracy. This applies not only to the keyed form of the test, but to the scoring stencil.
8. Organize the test so that it is possible to complete all the items within the alloted amount of time.

* Max D. Engelhart. "Improving Classroom Testing," *What Research Says to the Teacher*, No. 31, Department of Classroom Teachers, American Educational Research Association of the National Education Association, Washington, D.C., December, 1964.

9. If essay questions are involved, be sure to allow sufficient time for responses.
10. After tests have been scored, do an item analysis of the results.

A few more general suggestions refer to the matter of preparing a test well in advance of the date it is to be given and putting the test aside for a while and coming back to it at a later time to check for ambiguities or obscure meanings. It is also desirable to have someone who is knowledgeable in the field (a fellow teacher, perhaps) check and review the items for accuracy and possible ambiguities.

Using Test Results

There is more to testing than mere administration, scoring, and interpretation of scores to students. Teachers can learn a great deal from tests: (1) It is possible to analyze the extent to which students benefited from the learning experiences covered by the test; (2) a great deal can be learned by the nature of the questions the students were able to answer and the extent to which they answered them; and (3) much can be learned from the kinds of questions the students could not answer. Often the latter can provide insights into the shortcomings of the method used to present the materials.

It is always desirable to analyze test results. The following form adapted from Thorndike and Hagen illustrates the simplest form of item analysis for multiple-choice items.* A card of this type should be prepared for each item. The following is an easy item.

Item:
Ⓐ
B
C
D
E

	A	B	C	D	E
Upper 25%	10				
Middle 50%	17		1	2	
Lower 25%	5	1	1	3	

Alternately, if there were 50 items on a test and the highest score in a group of 100 students were 45 and the lowest score 10, the papers

* Robert L. Thorndike and Elizabeth Hagen. *Measurement and Evaluation in Psychology and Education*, John Wiley & Sons, Inc., New York, 1961, p. 90.

could be separated on the basis of the top 25 scores and the lowest 25 scores. Responses in each group are tallied to indicate item difficulty.

Item:	Upper	Lower
A	0	4
Ⓑ	20	10
C	3	6
D	0	3
E	2	2

This item is in the medium range of difficulty. The item is good from the standpoint of the fact that each of the choices was selected by at least one person in the lower group. If the majority of persons in the lower group select just one of the incorrect options, the other three incorrect options should be revised if the test is to be given again.

An item of middle-difficulty type should be included toward the middle of the test. It is best to start with some fairly easy items. The more difficult items should be reserved for the end of the test.

Flanagan has developed statistical tables to enable instructors and others to do accurate item analyses using upper and lower limits as follows: 29%, 27%, 37%, and 16%.*

Item analysis provides meaningful information for improving teaching; it can also improve capability to construct tests. Tests used in this way serve not only as testing instruments from the standpoint of determining the thoroughness and extent of student learning, they also serve as self-teaching tools for the instructor.

Testing the Test

Before decisions are made about the use of tests, they should be evaluated on the basis of three important factors: validity, reliability, and practicability. *Validity* refers to the extent to which a test measures that which we seek to measure, to the exclusion of other things. *Reliability* relates to the degree of accuracy and precision achieved by the test in measuring the specific factors it is designed to measure. *Practicability* refers to practical considerations such as time, cost, scoring convenience, and testing conditions required.†

Validity is the most important characteristic of a test. It is vital to know what the test measures so that later inferences can be made from the test scores. At times we are concerned with knowing how well a test measures student achievement; at times we want to know how well a test predicts behavior; and at still other times we may be interested in the

---

* John C. Flanagan, *Calculating Correlation Coefficients.* American Institutes for Research, Pittsburgh, 1962.
† Robert L. Thorndike and Elizabeth Hagen, *op. cit.*, pp. 160-63.

extent to which a test assesses a particular trait. For this reason it is important that the test user investigate the validity of the test in measuring the particular information he is seeking to measure.

Reliability is important from the standpoint of determining the preciseness of a test in measuring information or behavior. Estimates of reliability may be obtained in several ways; probably the most efficient and rigorous is to administer two equivalent forms of the test on two different occasions. By correlating results from the two administrations of the test, it is possible to obtain a reliability coefficient that shows any tendency for individuals to vary in their performance. Other measures of reliability involve administering the same test twice, or scoring on odd and even items and comparing the scores for the two halves. Any variations may be described by what is known as a standard error of measurement which shows the degree to which repetitions of testing may yield differences in scores. It is always desirable to interpret test scores in terms of the kinds of variation expressed in standard errors of measurement.

The practicability of using a test is the third basis for making decisions about the use of tests and is also an important one. Each test user knows best the situations surrounding his particular needs and the feasibility of undertaking the use of certain tests. Budgets, time limitations, lack of assistance in scoring great numbers of tests, and difficulties in administration can all affect decisions about tests. These are important points the test user must weigh when he explores the availability of various tests for his purposes.

Testing the test on the basis of the three criteria of validity, reliability, and practicability should keep the test user from making serious errors in choosing tests for use in his particular program.

Thorndike and Hagen* compiled a useful list of text and reference books which should be valuable to test users as sources of information about tests and testing. These in addition to their own very useful book on the subject should be reviewed by instructors in schools of nursing. This group of references should prove useful to nursing instructors whether they develop their own tests for classroom use, or whether they use nationally standardized tests.

Types of Tests

Short-answer tests can be teacher-made or can be chosen from a wide variety of standardized published tests (National League for Nursing). One advantage of standardized tests is that norms have been established and it is possible to compare students' scores with those made by comparable groups of students taking the same tests.

Short-answer, multiple-choice tests are sometimes criticized because

---

* *Ibid.*, p. 209.

they rely quite heavily on direct recall of information with little consideration to thought processes, judgments, or values. Some teachers believe
the students are favored because the correct answer is presented as one
of the choices, which the student may recognize rather than remember,
although it should be remembered that recognition is a form of recall.
Also, there is the factor of guessing. However, formulas have been developed to offset elevation in scores which may result from following
hunches or making lucky guesses.

The advantages of short-answer tests are: (1) they save time; (2) they
are simpler and faster to score; (3) they can be scored objectively; (4) they
can be standardized; (5) they provide instructors with a good deal of
basic information about what students have learned and where there
may be weaknesses; and (6) they provide a good basis for review. In
general, short-answer tests tend to be more popular than essay examinations.

Oral Tests
Oral examinations have been successfully used for many years. They
are still very much in use in daily classroom activities at all levels and
especially at the higher levels as final qualifying examinations for advanced
degrees. The oral examinations can range from quick, short questions or
quizzes to more formal, structured oral examinations administered by a
committee.

Some of the advantages are that students have an opportunity to
demonstrate capability to organize their thoughts quickly, to present points
in a logical fashion, and to express themselves orally. When examiners
are prepared to score responses in an objective manner, using checklists or
some type of rating form, oral testing can be quite useful in evaluating
student progress.

Questionnaires
Questionnaires can be successful in situations where the intent of the
test is to elicit reactions to a topic. Questionnaires can provide opportunities for students to express their ideas about the quality of instruction,
the materials presented, the learning experiences, the kinds of knowledge
they feel they have acquired, and the attitudes they have developed. If
care is taken in structuring the questionnaire, it is possible to overcome
tendencies toward vagueness or ambiguity on the part of the respondent.

Interviews
Interviews are a type of oral examination which has long been popular.
They may be staged between one interviewer and one interviewee, a group
of interviewers and one interviewee, or possibly one interviewer and a group
of interviewees. The greatest advantage of the interview is the degree of

flexibility it permits and the amount of spontaneity it can generate. Interviewers frequently use some type of checklist to note the behaviors they observe in addition to notations on the actual response made by the interviewee. In some cases interviewers take notes or use devices such as tape recorders, dictation discs, or similar equipment to record responses.

The relative disadvantages are considered to be (1) the possibility for the development of unfavorable interaction between interviewer and interviewee; (2) the tendency for the interviewee to become emotional because of strain or feelings of inadequacy or other problems; (3) the possibility of the introduction of extraneous or irrelevant matters during the course of the interview (the skilled interviewer must be able to cope with questions raised by the interviewee asking for clarification or amplification); (4) the interviewee may resent the note-taking; and (5) the interviewee may react unfavorably to the presence of recording devices and his responses may in some way reflect this uneasiness.

If the interviews are structured carefully and the interviewer is skillful in handling contingencies, it is often possible to use this technique successfully for evaluation purposes. Frequently, interviews can be staged in groups where interviewees write their answers. Again, depending on the materials to be covered and the skill of the interviewer, it is possible to get very desirable results for purposes of evaluation.

Checklists

In some forms of testing the student is given a written statement describing a problem, or he may be shown a display which has been set up to meet certain criteria, or he may be asked to view a drawing, a photograph, or a film strip. He is then presented with a checklist on which to indicate the presence or absence of certain characteristics or conditions. Checklists of this type should be carefully developed. There are several types. Some involve only a list to be checked by the examinee. This requires only a response to the presence or absence of certain conditions. A forced-choice checklist requires the student to arrive at a decision about a situation. Specific descriptive statements are presented. The examinee is forced to choose one from a series of equally appealing possibilities that have been set up on the basis of discrimination and validity for certain criteria.* In the job-rating situation, "Pairs of statements about job performance must be found where [they] express equally favorable or unfavorable things about a man, but with only one of the statements in each pair actually differentiating between the men known to differ in job performance."†

* Anne Anastasi. *Psychological Testing*, 2nd ed., The Macmillan Company, New York, 1961, p. 510.
† B. von Haller Gilmer (ed.). *Industrial Psychology*, McGraw-Hill Book Company, Inc., New York, 1961, p. 299.

Written Situation Tests

This type of test is a miniature "lifelike" situation in which a "case" or "problem" is described and used to determine how well the student can apply what she learned in the classroom and in the laboratory to practical problems. The situation is presented in written form. The examinee must solve or handle the problem by choosing from a list of possible solutions offered in multiple-choice form, or by writing the proposed solution to the problem in essay form listing the steps to be taken.

Since nursing students go on the unit in the hospital very early in their educational program, it is relatively simple for instructors to describe situations realistically. The solutions to the problem are offered by the student on the basis of her knowledge and experience or on the basis of the judgment she would use if confronted with certain emergencies. The instructor must take into consideration the level of the student. A beginning student should not be asked for solutions to advanced problems in nursing. Scoring is usually done on the basis of the number of critical points covered. This form of testing is widely used by standardizing agencies as well as by schools of nursing because it simulates the problem-solving situation on the ward. Cardew presents many of these situation problems in all aspects of nursing education.[*] A case is described in detail, including background information about the patient. The student is then given a series of multiple-choice questions about patient care.

Patient Study—The Disarming Patient[†]

Mr. Roberts, a 19-year-old service station attendant in a large metropolitan area, was admitted to the hospital one week ago. At that time, eight marijuana cigarettes and a small envelope of tiny white tablets were found concealed in the lining of his shaving kit. During this first week, he was friendly, congenial, and frequently offered to assist the nurses with other patients and with routine hospital activities. Some of the patients commented that Mr. Roberts had been sent to the ward to watch them because "he isn't crazy."

The social worker's history revealed the following: The father is a soft-spoken, kindly person who talks freely about himself but refers all questions about the home to his wife. The mother organizes information well and seems to have every detail at her fingertips. The patient has two older sisters, who are apparently happily married and who have no history of "nervous disorders." As a child, Mr. Roberts was frequently sick with "colds" and "stomach upsets." His sisters thought he was frail and often came to his rescue in any difficulty that arose in grade school. During high school, Mr. Roberts was still "frail" but his sisters had tired of making excuses for him and teased him about being a "sissy."

[*] Emily C. Cardew. *Study Guide for Clinical Nursing*, rev. ed., J. B. Lippincott Company, Philadelphia, 1961, pp. 493-95.
[†] Cardew, *loc. cit.*

Mr. Roberts' teacher often asked him what he would like to do when he finished high school. Mr. Roberts hadn't thought about this, but his mother had always wanted him to go to college and be a music teacher like her brother. The father thought that since Mr. Roberts was frail he should work on a farm so he could be out-of-doors more. Bitter family arguments over this conflict started before the patient began kindergarten.

When Mr. Roberts was in the second year of high school, his complaints of being "sick" ceased. However, the high-school principal reported to the family that Mr. Roberts missed two or three days of school each week. Although circumstances seemed to implicate the patient in several petty thefts which occurred at school, no definite proof was ever established. The sisters had also missed money from their purses and had accused their brother of taking it. The mother refused to believe these accusations. She frequently referred to the fact that her family had always been "well to do" and that her son could never do such a thing.

When Mr. Roberts finished high school, he secured a position in a loan company but was discharged after a few weeks because he forged a check for 20 dollars. The company did not press charges because the mother repaid the money. The mother blamed this incident on the fact that she had married a "working man with little get up" and that these characteristics in the boy must have come from his father's family.

When a circus came to town, Mr. Roberts secured a job collecting tickets. Without saying anything to his family, he left town with the circus group. After he had been gone for three weeks, the police contacted the family to say that Mr. Roberts had been jailed on a charge of driving while intoxicated and being involved in a traffic accident. The mother's attorney was able to get Mr. Roberts released because "he was so young." Mr. Roberts promised he would "be good" and found a job in a service station. In two weeks he again disappeared and was heard from when he was jailed on a disorderly conduct charge. The court sent him to the hospital for observation and diagnosis. After a Rorschach and various other psychological tests had been administered, Mr. Roberts was diagnosed as sociopathic personality with drug addiction and alcoholism.

QUESTIONS RELATING TO THE PATIENT STUDY
1. When Mr. Roberts was eight years old, the approval of the group most important to him probably was that of his
   a._____parents.
   b._____playmates.
   c._____sisters.
   d._____teachers.
2. The pattern most typical of Mr. Roberts' basic personality is that of
   a._____dependency.
   b._____depression.
   c._____independence.
   d._____repressed guilt.

3. The nurse can anticipate that developing rapport with Mr. Roberts will be established
   a._____with difficulty over a long period of time.
   b._____with difficulty within a few days.
   c._____without difficulty, but within a few days.
   d._____without difficulty over a period of weeks.
4. The nursing team should be firm, but kind and consistent in their nursing of Mr. Roberts because he
   a._____does not have a knowledge of the law.
   b._____has a strong, rigid supergo.
   c._____has an inflated concept of himself.
   d._____has never developed a realistic concept of the self.
5. The underlying reason for Mr. Roberts' not assuming social responsibility for his actions was that he
   a._____did not attend school regularly.
   b._____drank too much alcohol.
   c._____lacked a knowledge of the law.
   d._____none of the above.
6. One of the underlying etiologic factors in Mr. Roberts' illness was
   a._____alcohol addiction.
   b._____childhood experiences.
   c._____marijuana addiction.
   d._____organic lesions in the brain.
7. According to Cleckley, the dominant factor in Mr. Roberts' basic personality structure is characterized by a "weak"
   a._____id.
   b._____libido.
   c._____superego.
   d._____none of the above.
8. The main reason for the Rorschach test was to determine
   a._____intelligence.
   b._____reading comprehension.
   c._____vocabulary.
   d._____none of these.
9. Which of the following statements is applicable to Mr. Roberts' behavior?
   a._____Does not have a cause.
   b._____Is not motivated.
   c._____Was purposeful.
   d._____All of the above.

. . . .

A project undertaken by the staff of the American Institutes for Research involved the revision of the Medical Examination for Interns given by the National Board of Medical Examiners.* One of the types of tests

* Project conducted by the American Institutes for Research on the Development and Experimental Evaluation of an Improved Part III Examination for the National Board of Medical Examiners, 1959. (See list of critical requirements for interns and residents in Appendix I.)

used for this project involved the development of a film sequence emphasizing certain important aspects of patient examination and treatment. Following the showing of the film, examinees were given series of questions that they were to answer based on the problems presented in the film.

One of the advantages to this type of test is that the examinee does not have to imagine the situation based on what he has read about the problem. He is presented with a visual enactment of the problem which makes it possible to convey interaction of the doctor and the patient, the doctor and other personnel, and other factors which are somewhat difficult, if not almost impossible, to convey in a written situation problem.

Another advantage is the standardized problem the film presents. No aspect of the situation is left to the varied interpretations which result when different people read a description of an examination or a treatment. The film presents the same situation to everyone at the same time. The judgments of the students about what they have seen in the film provide the basis for decisions about the way in which they answer the questions on the test.

Observational Situation Tests

Another type of situation test is one we will call Critical Factor Performance Test, or the Observational Situation Test, in which the student actively participates in the action required to handle the problem. Nursing lends itself very well to this type of test because students actually have opportunities to work in real-life situations involving real patients with real problems; there is no need for simulation. Although patients' problems may not be exactly alike, it is possible to select those whose problems are sufficiently similar that the testing situations are comparable. The Critical Factor Performance Test provides an opportunity to observe the student in action, demonstrating what she has learned in the way of patient care and her approach to solving problems. The observer is able to record behaviors that are real, not simply an indication of what the student *might* do, but what she actually *does* do when confronted by a problem situation.

Scoring on this type of test can be done in several ways: behavior checklists can be used similar to the one constructed by Gorham, Lichtenstein, and Marchese;* rating sheets also can be used. The critical incident technique is most useful in this type of test because the observer is not forced to watch for or check certain types of behaviors according to a specified checklist; the observer records critical incidents as they occur. There is no need to make a judgment about degrees of quality; incidents are effective or ineffective, depending on the significance of the outcome. If the student demonstrates that she is able to carry out the procedure

* William A. Gorham, Stanley Lichtenstein, and Angeline C. Marchese. *Specific Nursing Behaviors Related to Patient Care and Improvement: Measuring Nursing Performance*, American Institutes for Research, Washington, D.C., 1959, D-1.

and provide effective care to the patient, an effective incident is recorded in the appropriate category of behavior.

Performance tests of this type can be most useful if it is possible to achieve comparable testing situations and if observers have been trained to observe critical incidents of behavior relevant to the problem.

Example of *Critical Factor Performance Test Item*

The situation takes place in the emergency room of a hospital. The student nurse involved is the examinee. Actors include a "mother" who brings in an "infant" who is ill, a resident physician, and a staff nurse. (Clock on the wall indicates time is 2:45 P.M. It should take about 15 minutes for the problem to take place. Clock will then show 3:00 P.M.)

Problem

A mother brings an infant (a doll) to the emergency room. She explains in distraught fashion that the infant is choking and cannot stop. The resident takes the child and asks the mother to go into the waiting room (mother leaves the room). The resident then instructs the student to assist him by holding the child's arms gently away from the chest as the resident examines him. The baby (doll) is lying on a table and the resident works with the child to relieve the convulsion. The resident comments that the convulsion is subsiding and that the child is "all right." He directs the student to attend the child as he writes his orders. At that point a staff nurse comes in and the resident says, "Good, now that you're here, you can take over. I think we will keep the child here overnight. Will you take care of getting him ready." (To the student) "Thanks, I guess that's it. Miss Jordan is here now, so you may leave. See you tomorrow."

From this point on, the student (examinee) makes her decisions about next steps. She has been relieved by the staff nurse, the time is 3:00 P.M. Technically, she is free to go off duty. The mother is still in the waiting room, which is across from the emergency room. The student has been relieved and may go.

Possibilities

1. The student might say she will stay for a few minutes in case she can help.
2. She could tell the staff nurse that she will see her tomorrow and at that point leave the emergency room.
3. She may leave the emergency room and go to the waiting room where the mother is waiting. She may assure the mother that the child is over the choking spell and appears to be much improved. She may tell the mother that the resident will be over in a few minutes to talk with her about the baby's condition and what should be done. She

should not, however, provide any information about the diagnosis. She should merely reassure the mother.

The most effective behavior is that in 3 since this is an opportunity for interpersonal relations in comforting the worried mother. If the student recalls that the mother is waiting and perceives the need to reassure her about the infant's condition, this would be an effective behavior on the part of the student in assuming her responsibility toward the family.

Nothing during the action of the problem directs the student to go out to reassure the mother. The student must think of this on her own and must initiate the action. She could mention to the resident and the staff nurse that she will do this. If she does, they should make some indication that this would be a good idea. The student provides all the initiating action in approaching the mother. The mother can interact by continuing to show concern, but she does not say anything until the student finishes.

One good way to standardize the testing situation is to present the problem using moving pictures plus student participants. It is possible to record the situation on film including all appropriate information about actions leading up to the problem. The film stops just short of the solution or the necessary action to provide patient care. The student then takes over and demonstrates how she would go about solving the problem or giving the needed patient care.

A great deal of success can be achieved if video tape is used to record the behavior of the student. The advantage is that it can be played back to the student, showing her exactly how she behaved. The playback can be accompanied by comments from the instructor relative to the effectiveness or ineffectiveness of the behavior.

The disadvantage might be the cost of this type of testing. However, the benefits are sufficient to warrant the expenditure for the equipment to provide this type of testing situation at least for some aspects of the education program. New types of video tape are available that are relatively inexpensive and serve adequately for purposes of quick playback of action.

National agencies also have movie situations that can be used for testing purposes. These can be used repeatedly for testing students either in groups or individually. An ideal method for the filmed situation is to use one requiring the action of a nursing team to handle the problem. Students can be assigned responsibilities, and the observer can note the effectiveness or ineffectiveness with which each student accepts and carries out her duties in the team situation.

Other advantages in using Critical Factor Performance tests are: (1) they test student ability to choose from alternate solutions; (2) they provide opportunities for students to demonstrate certain behavioral traits in handling problems or emergencies that cannot be demonstrated on written tests; (3) they create situations in which the student can demonstrate ability to interact with a patient; (4) they help students to demonstrate ability to interact with others on the health team, including doctors, supervisors, head nurses, ancillary personnel; and (5) the checklists used for scoring provide valuable feedback to the instructor and the student.

Observers of performance on tests of this type should be provided with criteria and checklists or rating forms on which to record observations.

Area A

Contributing to medical treatment of patient

	1	2	3	4	5
Effective behaviors					
Reminded doctor about scheduled procedures					
Contacted doctor for enema or laxative order					
Assembled equipment in anticipation of needs					
Checked on-going treatment periodically					
Prevented interruptions in on-going procedure					
Ineffective behaviors					
Used inadequate substitutes for ordered treatments					
Delayed following stat orders					
Omitted giving medication					
Made error in dosage					
Forgot to report patient's symptoms					
Gave treatment at incorrect time					

Figure 5   Sample of a checklist.

Profile of Performance of the General Duty Nurse

In your experience as a nurse, you have at times observed the strong and weak points of general duty nurses. You may have said of a nurse, "She is very skillful in giving treatments, but she doesn't know how to get along with patients." or, "She really knows how to make a patient comfortable, but she isn't sure of how to carry out procedures." These judgments are based on your day-to-day observations of the nurse.

Because of your close working relations with your co-workers, you are in an especially good position to tell how the general duty nurses on your unit perform in each of five nursing care areas. On this form, we are not concerned with how effective a nurse is in relation to other nurses; we are concerned about her relative performance in each of the areas. For example, the nurse may be the best nurse on the unit, but she is probably not equally effective in each of the five areas. It is more likely that she is better in one or two of the areas than she is in others. In order words, a profile of a given nurse's performance in the five areas would show that she is strong in some areas and less strong in others.

How to Complete the Form

1.   Fill out a profile sheet for each of the nurses on your ward. If you are a general duty nurse, fill out one on yourself, also.

2.   Enter the nurse's name and your own name in the spaces provided. This information will be confidential. Names are necessary only for purposes of comparing various data obtained.

3.   Read the brief descriptions of the five nursing care areas.

4.   Divide 100 points among the five areas, according to how strong you think the nurse is in each area. You may do this by checking the appropriate point on the scale under each area.

5.   Enter in the sum column for each area the number of points corresponding to the point you have checked on the scale. You should have 5 numbers in this column. Be sure they total 100.

Figure 6A   (From J. Wayne Wrightstone *et al. Evaluation in Modern Education*, American Book Co., New York, 1956.)

Observers should be trained to make objective judgments. Reputation and "halo" factors should be reduced or, better still, eliminated.

Checklists

These are lists of selected words, phrases, or sentences. The observer makes a check mark noting the presence or the absence of characteristics or of behavior. Behavior checklists are extremely useful to instructors in scoring performance on oral presentation, on laboratory performance, on critical factor performance tests, or on performance on the unit. Checklists have numerous advantages. (1) They provide a profile of student behavior which the instructor can analyze and discuss with the student. (2) They offer insights into problem areas. (3) They may be useful in devising ways for correcting deficiencies, overcoming weaknesses, and in revising

Profile of Performance

Nurse you are describing _____   Your name _____   Date _____

Ward _____

Area I	Area II	Area III	Area IV	Area V
Providing psychological care to patients - explaining treatments, procedures, and condition; teaching self-care; providing emotional support.	Providing physical care to patients - promoting comfort, hygiene, and safety; attending to the patient's physical and rehabilitation needs.	Assisting with medical care - giving medicines and treatments; observing and reporting; acting appropriately in emergency and p. r. n. situations; handling equipment.	Arranging management details - instructing and supervising auxiliary personnel; planning and scheduling nursing care; maintaining general supplies; supervising visitors.	Personal characteristics - behaving in a warm and friendly manner; being attentive and tactful; being pleasant under pressure; behaving in a professional manner

Sum

I _____
II _____
III _____
IV _____
V _____

Total 100

Figure 6B   (From J. Wayne Wrightstone et al. *Evaluation in Modern Education,* American Book Co., New York, 1956.)

teaching to compensate for any oversights observed. (4) Students can benefit from the use of checklists because it is possible to learn what kinds of behaviors will be expected for satisfactory or acceptable performance; they help to establish goals of behavior toward which students can work. (5) Checklists reduce observer subjectivity because less judgment is required; there is less need to assess the quality since the observer uses a series of checks denoting the presence or absence of behavior.

The possible disadvantages are that observers may tend to go down the list with little regard for the facts. Also, if students have an opportunity to study checklists, they may tend to make efforts to demonstrate the desirable behaviors just for the purpose of the test. However, this is usually not too much of a problem in nursing because students can be presented with enough real problems to provide ample opportunity to demonstrate whether they are "acting" to get a good score, or whether they are performing nursing duties in a competent manner and administering care that will result in the utmost benefit to the patient.

Checklists can be extremely useful not only in scoring performance and behavior but also for purposes of curriculum planning. Students can use checklists to indicate their reactions to certain factors about the courses or learning experiences they have had. Such lists help teachers to learn a great deal about student attitude toward courses, and whether certain instruction is regarded as adequate. If checklists are constructed skillfully enough, it should be possible to have students indicate what shortcomings they believe exist in the curriculum.

Other checklists involve evaluation on procedural tasks (Fig. 7).

Rating Scales

One very popular type of evaluation tool is the rating scale which is somewhat similar to the checklist. The rating scale is used to describe observations of performance. Like the checklist, it also involves words, phrases, sentences, or descriptive paragraphs to guide the observer. However, rating scales have an added feature; they involve judgments as to quantity or quality. For example, the ratings might range from *exceptional, outstanding,* or *excellent* at the higher end of the scale to *unsatisfactory, poor,* or *incapable of doing the job* at the bottom. There may be other points on the continuum; the ratings might be in the form of number values, or the observer may be asked to record whether a behavior occurs "always," "frequently," "fairly often," "sometimes," or "never." This leaves rating to the observer.

In the project to investigate specific nursing behavior related to patient care* a forced-distribution rating scale was designed to obtain evaluations of over-all performance as well as performance in specific areas. This form makes it possible to compare performance from one person to another, from one group to another, and also to compare the performance of a single

* Gorham, *et al., loc. cit.*

nurse in several areas. The form consisted of 50 statements describing behavior grouped into five major categories. The rater was asked to compare performance observed using the following scale:

Problem: Improving Patient's Adjustment to Hospitalization or Illness
—Preparing Patient Psychologically for Treatment

Top 20%   Next 20%   Next 20%   Next 20%   Low 20%

This type of scale is better than a simple graphic scale because it forces the rater to distribute ratings of individuals over the entire rating scale rather than rate everyone about the same and at the same point in the scale (usually the higher end).

Grading on a curve is one common example of a forced distribution. Distributing grades in this way usually results in a few A's at the high end and a few E's or F's at the lower end, with a greater concentration of B's and D's, and the greatest number being graded as C's. The curve refers to the normal curve of distribution which assumes that traits or abilities of individuals tend to be distributed symmetrically around some quantitative mean, and that most people fall fairly close to the mean. This is the assumption inherent in most of the statistical techniques currently in use. It is further assumed that any given group of individuals is fairly representative of all persons in whom we are interested.

A forced distribution has several advantages. (1) It makes the rater discriminate among the individuals she is rating. A rating scale on which most individuals are rated at about the same point has little or no value. (2) Forced distributions reduce the tendency of some raters to rate higher or lower on all people than other raters. (3) When forced distributions are used, it is possible to compare persons on the same scale and also to combine them. (4) The forced distribution results in a more normal distribution. For example, if one teacher of a course in ward relationships gives only one A while a second teacher gives five A's, it is difficult to make comparisons of the relative achievement in each of the classes. However, if both teachers were forced to make a more normal distribution of A's, the comparison would be considerably easier. Many other factors are involved, of course, but this example is based on two groups of comparable ability, the same number of students, and the same kinds of teaching materials and unit outlines. Using forced distributions of grades in this type of situation should yield more comparable sets of grades than other kinds of rating approaches.

Open-end rating scales represent another type of rating device. No numerical grading is done on these scales. The rater is presented with a

CHECKLIST OF STUDENT REACTIONS IN FINDING AN OBJECT UNDER THE MICROSCOPE

Student's name_____   Time begun_____

Section _____   Time finished _____

Date_____   Time consumed _____

DIRECTIONS

On the microscope table are a microscope, yeast culture, or other suitable material, slides, covers, cloth, and lens paper. Direct the student to find a cell or other object under the microscope and show it to you. Time him in seconds from the time he receives the directions. Trace his actions by placing a figure 1 after his first action, a figure 2 after his second action, and so on in the order of his performance. Characterize his behavior and his mount by checking appropriate terms from the lists given below.

Add any additional comments in the blank on this page. In summarizing the student's actions the instructor may wish to suggest skills in which the student should receive additional training by checking the appropriate items in the list of skills in which student needs further training.

STUDENT'S ACTIONS	SEQUENCE OF ACTIONS	STUDENT'S ACTIONS	SEQUENCE OF ACTIONS
a. Takes slide	_____	o. Places slide on stage	_____
b. Wipes slide with lens paper	_____	p. Looks through eyepiece with right eye	_____
c. Wipes slide with cloth	_____	q. Looks through eyepiece with left eye	_____
d. Wipes slide with finger	_____	r. Turns to objective of lowest power	_____
e. Moves bottle of culture along the table	_____	s. Turns to low-power objective	_____
f. Places drop or two of culture on slide	_____	t. Turns to high-power objective	_____
g. Adds more culture	_____	u. Holds one eye closed	_____
h. Adds few drops of water	_____	v. Looks for light	_____
i. Hunts for cover glasses	_____	w. Adjusts concave mirror	_____
j. Wipes cover glass with lens paper	_____	x. Adjusts plane mirror	_____
k. Wipes cover with cloth	_____	y. Adjusts diaphragm	_____
l. Wipes cover with finger	_____	z. Does not touch diaphragm	_____
m. Adjusts cover with finger	_____		
n. Wipes off surplus fluid	_____		

Figure 7

STUDENT'S ACTION	SEQUENCE OF ACTIONS		STUDENT'S ACTION	SEQUENCE OF ACTIONS
aa. With eye at eyepiece turns down coarse adjustment	_____		NOTICEABLE CHARACTERISTICS OF STUDENT'S BEHAVIOR	
ab. Breaks cover glass	_____		a. Awkward in movements	_____
ac. Breaks slide	_____		b. Obviously dexterous in movements	_____
ad. With eye away from eyepiece turns down coarse adjustment	_____		c. Slow and deliberate	_____
			d. Very rapid	_____
ae. Turns up coarse adjustment a great distance	_____		e. Finger tremble	_____
af. With eye at eyepiece turns down fine adjustment a great distance	_____		f. Obviously perturbed	_____
			g. Does not take work seriously	_____
			h. Obviously angry	_____
ag. With eye away from eyepiece turns down fine adjustment a great distance	_____		i. Unable to work without specific directions	_____
ah. Turns up fine adjustment screw a great distance	_____		j. Obviously satisfied with his unsuccessful efforts	_____
ai. Turns fine adjustment screw a few turns	_____		CHARACTERIZATIONS OF THE STUDENT'S MOUNT	
aj. Removes slide from stage	_____		a. Poor light	_____
ak. Wipes objective with lens paper	_____		b. Poor focus	_____
al. Wipes objective with cloth	_____		c. Excellent mount	_____
am. Wipes objective with finger	_____		d. Good mount	_____
an. Wipes eyepiece with lens paper	_____		e. Fair mount	_____
			f. Poor mount	_____
ao. Wipes eyepiece with cloth	_____		g. Very poor mount	_____
ap. Wipes eyepiece with finger	_____		h. Nothing in view but a thread in his eyepiece	_____
aq. Makes another mount	_____			
ar. Takes another microscope	_____		i. Something on objective	_____
as. Finds object	_____		j. Smeared lens	_____
at. Pauses for an interval	_____		k. Unable to find object	_____
au. Asks, "What do you want me to do?"	_____		SKILLS IN WHICH STUDENT NEEDS FURTHER TRAINING	
av. Asks whether to use high power	_____		a. In cleaning objective	_____
aw. Says, "I'm satisfied"	_____		b. In cleaning eyepiece	_____
ax. Says that the mount is all right for his eye	_____		c. In focusing low power	_____
			d. In focusing high power	_____
ay. Says he cannot do it	_____		e. In adjusting mirror	_____
az. Told to start a new mount	_____		f. In using diaphragm	_____
aaa. Directed to find object under low power	_____		g. In keeping both eyes open	_____
aab. Directed to find object under high power	_____		h. In protecting slide and objective from breaking by careless focusing	_____

Figure 7 (concluded)

list of behaviors considered to be either desirable or undesirable for the particular job. The rater is to assess the quality of performance or the extent to which specific behaviors were present or absent. The raters write in their comments rather than using percentage points or letters to indicate their ratings. The rater comments on this type of scale often range from a broad generalization such as "good in this area" or "fine" to long, descriptive paragraphs about specific details of performance. The disadvantage of this type of scale is that too much is left to the judgment of the rater. More adept raters will naturally be able to use this kind of scale more effectively. However, if the rater is not skilled in making evaluations, or if he is "too busy with other things and wants to get ratings out of his way," there might be a tendency to skim over the lists of behaviors in a haphazard manner, or to rely too heavily on memory, judgment, or reputation rather than to take the necessary time to record ratings based on actual observation. Another problem is that raters often tend to disagree on what is important. Or, they tend to disagree on the meanings of the descriptive terms used. If this is the case, it is difficult to quantify the ratings. Open-end scales leave margin for error in judgment and are often regarded as being the least effective of the tools used to evaluate performance. When there is too much latitude left to the judgment of the rater, the purpose of evaluation can be defeated.

Rothney listed a number of reasons that ratings cannot always be regarded as ideal evaluation instruments. He states:

> . . . ratings may be definitely harmful since research has shown that among their other limitations they a) suggest that certain characteristics are equally desirable in equal amounts for all individuals at all times; b) encourage generalization about a pupil's charactertistics beyond what was actually observed by the rater; c) encourage the making of comparisons of pupils who are quite different and who have had unequal environmental opportunities; d) assume that the teacher can observe behavior, such as cooperation, sort it into units on a scale, and allot values to it; e) suffer from "halo" effect, that is, the teachers who rates a pupil high in one characteristic tends to rate him high in others or vice versa; and f) usually suffer from inadequate definition of the terms to be rated so that what is satisfactory to one person may be very unsatisfactory to another.*

Rothney contends:

> . . . it is unrealistic and unwise to try to place pupils on the same scale without considering their unique circumstances and situations.†

* John W. M. Rothney. "Evaluating and Reporting Pupil Progress," *What Research Says to the Teacher*, American Educational Research Association of the National Education Association, Washington, D.C., 1955, p. 16.
† *Ibid.*, p. 17.

There is constant danger in using rating sheets because raters try to "make" the behaviors observed fit the limitations of the checklist without considering the degree of behavior manifested and the individual differences in the people being rated.

Thorndike and Hagen cite a number of the problems encountered in the use of rating scales. They call attention to—

> . . . at least two sets of circumstances that may impair the integrity of a set of ratings: 1) The rater may be unwilling to take the trouble that is called for by the appraisal procedure; and 2) The rater may identify with the person rated to such an extent that he is unwilling to make a rating that will hurt him.*

In support of the first factor mentioned above is the problem of the rater's not being convinced of the importance of the rating procedures; therefore, he is unwilling to devote the time or the effort to giving an unbiased rating to all the students in a class. On the other hand, the rater himself may have feelings of insecurity and tend to identify with the student to the extent that he finds it impossible to give an unbiased rating of performance. In military situations, for example, the obligation of the officer is to keep up the morale of his men. If an officer becomes known as a "tough" rater, the general morale of the unit may reflect the problem. The officer who may want to make his unit look good on the record may tend to rate his men a little on the "high" side to achieve this. Thorndike and Hagen cite situations during the last war when—

> . . . the typical rating, accounting for a very large proportion of the ratings given, was "excellent." "Very good" became an expression of marked dissatisfaction, while a rating of "satisfactory" was reserved for someone to be transferred at the first opportunity.†

Other problems involve a hesitancy on the part of a rater to condemn someone by a low rating because this might have some bearing on whether or not that person is maintained on the staff or in the school. Still another difficulty in using rating scales is the inconsistency in interpretating various intervals along the continuum—how "outstanding" must a nurse be to be rated as "outstanding?" Conversely, what constitutes a rating of "unsatisfactory" performance? Often a teacher sets a very high standard and feels that no one is truly "outstanding." On the other hand, some teachers are concerned with granting recognition to promote high morale and, therefore, will give a rating of "outstanding" for what some would consider as merely "good" performance.

---

* Robert L. Thorndike and Elizabeth Hagen. *Measurement and Evaluation in Psychology and Education,* John Wiley & Sons, Inc., New York, 1961, p. 355.
† *Ibid.,* p. 356.

Reliability of ratings tends to increase when the number of raters increases. Often when only one person is responsible for an individual, the rating on a student may be too high because the rater has heard that this student is "good," and she doesn't want her ratings to disagree with what others think. This is another example of the "halo effect"—a situation in which the rater is influenced by prior knowledge about the individual. Halo effects can exist in situations where the individual seems to be able "to do everything well;" or conversely there may be a feeling on the part of the rater that the individual "can't do anything right." Raters are frequently influenced, whether consciously or unconsciously, by halo effects. Reputation can also be a factor.

Thorndike and Hagen state that ratings are greatly improved when the rater is given a number of specific descriptions of behavior rather than a long list of traits, because specificity tends to reduce ambiguity.* They caution, however, that lengthy lists of behaviors may cause confusion. The lists are most effective when the judgment to be made is quite simple, and where some provision is made for organizing and summarizing rater judgments.

Another type of rating scale requires students to rate one another. This is sometimes known as "peer rating" or "buddy rating." If this procedure is used, the student should be given an opportunity to learn what is expected in the rating situation and should be "briefed" on the meanings of the terms used and the scope of each interval on the rating scale. Peer ratings can be useful. However, here again there is the danger of the influence of halo effects or the tendency of friends to rate one another a little higher because of their friendship, or conversely, for those who don't get along well to underrate some of their peers because of a personal bias.

Forced-Choice Rating Scales

This method tends to offset the disadvantages in other rating scales by making it less possible for the rater to control the results. The rater is presented with pairs or a series of three, four, or even five choices, all of which tend to be equally favorable or appealing, or all of which are equally unappealing or negative. Sometimes there are two favorable and two unfavorable, or there can be a series of three, and the rater must choose the most appealing or the least. The rater is forced to choose one statement from each pair or from the tetrad or pentad. The forced-choice scale—

> . . . requires two principal types of information regarding each descriptive phrase, vis., its social desirability or "preference index" and its empirical validity or "discriminative index." The latter may be determined on the basis of any specific criterion the inventory is designed to predict.

* Thorndike and Hagen, *op. cit.*, p. 362.

. . . Social desirability can be found by having the items rated for this variable by a representative group, or by ascertaining the frequency with which the item is endorsed in self-descriptions.*

Advantages of this technique are that it leaves less judgment to the bias of the rater and it involves less ambiguity than the "yes-no" or "true-false" types of ratings, or the ratings involving terms that require interpretation, such as "excellent," "good," or "fair."

Rating scales of the forced-choice type have been used for rating performance. It has been found that they tend to reduce (although they do not entirely eliminate) the bias of the rater. The rater is forced to make the choice not knowing which item is most discriminating. This kind of a rating scale is usually regarded as somewhat less effective when used by a rater than when used for self-rating purposes.†

An example of the use of a forced-choice type of profile for rating the performance of nurses is shown in Figure 8.

Self-Rating

Rating scales are sometimes used for self-rating. The scales can be graphic, descriptive, forced-choice, numerical, or other types. In this situation students are presented with the choices on the rating scale and are asked to rate themselves on the various behaviors listed. This, too, can be heavily influenced by personal tendencies of the raters in underestimating or over-estimating their own capabilities or achievements. Some students will rate themselves high, despite their own realization of a lack in a particular area, to make their rating sheet "look good" in comparison to others. There are students whose feelings of insecurity may make them rate their own performance as borderline, average, or even unsatisfactory because they cannot be completely objective in evaluating themselves. Much of the success of self-rating programs depends upon the preliminary training of the students to recognize their own strengths and weaknesses and to be objective in rating their own performance. When objectivity in self-rating can be achieved, this procedure can prove useful.

Ranking

At times raters are asked to "rank" subordinates, giving them a numerical position with relation to their peers in the group. This will frequently resolve some of the problems encountered when a rater is influenced by halo effects or reputation where certain individuals are concerned. Ranking involves placing students in an order, taking into consideration degrees of difference between individuals. When ranking

* Anne Anastasi. *Psychological Testing*, 2nd ed., The Macmillan Company, New York, 1961, p. 511.
† *Ibid.*, pp. 514-15.

134

Name of the nurse being described _____

Name of the nurse completing the form _____

Date _____

Instructions

This form consists of 50 pairs of statements describing things that a general duty nurse may do. In each of the pairs in Part I, you are asked to check the one statement which is most typical of the usual performance of the nurse you are describing. In some pairs, it may be difficult to make a choice, because both of the statements may seem to describe the nurse. However, you will be giving a more revealing picture of the nurse when you indicate only one statement as most typical of her. It is also very important that you check one statement in every pair in order to give a complete picture of the nurse's performance.

Part I

1. Overcomes resistance to self-care. _____
   Instructs patients in personal care. _____

2. Informs doctors about errors in orders. _____
   Catches disagreement between charts and medicine cards. _____

3. Uses proper equipment in treatments. _____
   Assembles equipment in anticipation of needs. _____

4. Reduces noise in patients' environment. _____
   Maintains neatness of patients' environment. _____

5. Orders medications from pharmacy promptly. _____
   Forces fluids when ordered. _____

6. Keeps upsetting visitors from patients. _____
   Limits visiting time to prevent patient fatigue. _____

7. Bathes patients promptly. _____
   Helps others in movement of patients. _____

8. Uncovers pertinent information in patient's history. _____
   Questions patients about their symptoms. _____

9. Measures fluid intakes and outputs accurately. _____
   Observes patients for side-effects of drugs. _____

Figure 8 Forced-choice rating scale.

10. Reassures patients about the quality of hospital care. _____
    Provides patients with distracting activities. _____

11. Takes initiative in health teaching. _____
    Demonstrates self-care procedures. _____

12. Checks accuracy of requisition slips. _____
    Prepares medications rapidly. _____

13. Informs doctors about patients' needs. _____
    Reports patients' reactions to medication. _____

14. Contacts other hospital departments for patients. _____
    Calls outside agencies to reduce patients' expenses. _____

15. Checks on adequacy of drugs on hand. _____
    Prepares equipment for physicians' use. _____

16. Talks with patients to relax them. _____
    Teaches patients to observe their reactions. _____

17. Promptly notifies physicians of new admissions. _____
    Reminds doctors about scheduled procedures. _____

18. Gives treatments in appropriate order. _____
    Schedules treatments to minimize delays. _____

19. Checks adequacy of food trays. _____
    Massages patients to make them comfortable. _____

20. Tells patients about similar successful treatments. _____
    Explains necessity for exercises. _____

21. Treats bed sores. _____
    Encourages exercises for rehabilitation. _____

22. Contacts social workers for patients. _____
    Refers patients for rehabilitation purposes. _____

23. Explains importance of rest and relaxation. _____
    Gives needed care despite patients' resistance. _____

24. Provides patients with pamphlets on condition. _____
    Shows patients how to overcome physical defects. _____

25. Explains necessity for diagnostic procedures. _____
    Explains reasons for patients' symptoms. _____

Figure 8 (concluded)

is required, the observer must finally admit that one student surpasses another, and that they are not all "very good" or "above average," or conversely, they are not all just average or below.*

When rating scales or checklists are to be used for evaluation, the instruments should be developed with care so that they will be as effective as possible. The head nurse, or the instructor, should have valuable contributions to a list of behaviors for use in a rating scale. Behaviors should include those appropriate for the tasks to be evaluated. The lists of behaviors should be developed by several people in order to reduce the possibility of narrowness of scope which a single contributor might have. Another advantage in having several people involved is that the aims and purposes of the rating tool or checklist become more clearly understood by the group. In some cases it is desirable to seek expert assistance for additional unbiased information.

Another way to identify appropriate behaviors for a rating scale or checklist is to use task performance information and descriptions or to use critical incidents. The critical incident technique is particularly useful because it provides examples of actual behavior on the job, noted and recorded on the basis of firsthand observation. An analysis of critical incidents should yield a useful set of behaviors for a rating scale or checklist.

The important points to remember in constructing checklists or rating scales is the identification and clear-cut description of major behavior areas. Ambiguity of major headings can lead to confusion. Sometimes there is too much overlap from one category to another, or subcategories may be too closely related. As far as possible this overlap and duplication should be reduced or eliminated. After the scales have been developed and tried out, they should be put into use, with an adequate number of qualified raters competent to make appropriate judgments.

The main disadvantage to ranking is that it is difficult to present the amount of difference that exists between each interval of the ranking scale. For example, if scores on a test are rank-ordered and presented in that order, it is difficult to tell the extent to which one person excelled another in performance. Micheels and Karnes illustrate this point as follows:†

	Score		*Rank Order*	
Difference of	⎰ 96	1 ⎱	Difference of 1 point	
1 point in	⎱ 95	2 ⎰	in rank order	
score				
Difference of	⎰ 94	3 ⎱	Difference of 1 point	
13 points in	⎱ 81	4 ⎰	in rank order	
score				

* Thorndike and Hagen, *op. cit.*, pp. 371-72.
† William J. Micheels and M. Ray Karnes. *Measuring Educational Achievement*, McGraw-Hill Series in Education, New York, 1950, p. 422.

This same type of problem also can exist in ranking performance because the interval between the quality of the performance of one person as compared with another may show as one point on the ranking scale, yet there could be quite a range between the performance of the two persons. Rankings can be useful to show relative standings of persons in a group when an explanation is presented to clarify the degrees of difference that exist from one interval on the ranking scale to another.

OBSERVATIONAL TECHNIQUES

One of the very oldest methods for evaluating performance is by direct observation of performance. Notations of the actions a person goes through in doing a job and the behaviors that are manifest in those actions has been the basis for evaluation of performance since ancient days. Direct observation is still regarded as the most effective means for objective evaluation. The recording of observations can be handled in a variety of ways.

Anecdotal Notes

Probably the first record of observations was made in the form of anecdotal notes. They consisted of informal descriptions of observations made on the behavior and activities of subjects or students. There are seldom any specific instructions to follow, the observer just makes notes of what he observes, including enough detail to convey information. Anecdotal notes can be quite cryptic, they can be mere jottings, or they can be small descriptive paragraphs. They often run the gamut from terse statements of critical factors to rather ambiguous descriptions. At times they contain little more than opinions, depending on the skill of the observer in separating factual information from bias or personal judgment.

Thorndike and Hagan cite five features of a good anecdotal note or record.* To be effective and useful, an anecdote should—

1. Contain a good, accurate description of a specific event;
2. Include sufficient description to give the event meaning;
3. Contain a separate notation if some interpretation or evaluation is made;
4. Describe an event relating the performance of the person to others on the staff;
5. Relate an event representative of typical behavior for the student, or significantly different from usual behavior. Departure from typical behavior should be noted. Improvement of past behavior also should be noted.

A common problem in anecdotal note recording is that the notes often

* Thorndike and Hagen, *op. cit.*, p. 415.

include evaluation as opposed to straight recording of facts. The note may represent an interpretation of the behavior rather than a direct account of it.

Some observers have difficulty deciding what to record on an anecdotal note. Observers should make it a practice to record observations of behavior that are significantly important to shed some light on various aspects of student development, such as interaction with others, attitudes, and demonstration of the use of knowledges and skills. Anecdotal notes are not intended to measure academic proficiency, to estimate tendencies toward creativity, or to make estimates of intellectual abilities—standardized objective tests do a much better job in these areas. When measures of academic achievement are desired, teachers should use tests designed for this purpose. Anecdotal notes are intended to serve as a record of events that occurred during a particular period of performance. Anecdotal notes that are vague or ambiguous or that include too much detail are not very useful.

The quality of anecdotal notes often can depend on the mood of the observer. For example, consider the following note on Miss McNeilly:

She consistently monopolizes ward conference time. Brings up irrelevant issues. Confuses other students and disrupts class. Introduces personal problems to divert the attention of others to herself. She is a menace to the group.

What does this contribute to (1) insight into the behavior of Miss McNeilly or (2) information that can be used by other instructors?

First, the statement "consistently monopolizes" is a matter of judgment or opinion. It is impossible to determine from this note whether Miss McNeilly behaved in this way for the first time, the fourth time, or the fifth time. However, it could be inferred that the behavior had occurred before. Does "monopolizing" imply taking over the entire session, part of it, or perhaps just discussion time? The note alludes to "irrelevant" issues. Are these matters that students would also agree are irrelevant? Perhaps the student felt they were relevant. How can it be determined that Miss McNeilly's purpose was to direct attention toward herself? She may or may not consciously have acted in this way. It is possible that, if Miss NcNeilly is attempting to deal with a very difficult personal problem, her behavior was an indication of the need for help. The use of the term "menace" does not add to the accuracy of the note; it is further evidence of the bias of the observer. It is possible that she is a "menace" to the instructor only, and that the class does not react in this way to Miss McNeilly. In any case, this is not the type of anecdotal note that is of value in considering the effectiveness or ineffectiveness of Miss McNeilly's performance.

How could this note be improved? Consider the following:

On Oct. 10, Miss McNeilly interrupted ward conference by speaking out four times to ask questions or raise points that did not deal with the condition of the patients. She also took class time to present two personal problems that could have been discussed in a private conference with the instructor after class.

What are the distinguishing features about the second note? First, it contains a date. This makes it possible to fix the time when the behavior occurred. In this instance it occurred during the seventh week of the semester Miss McNeilly entered nursing school. For most students this would have been sufficient time to adjust to appropriate behavior. The revised note also cites the number of times interruptions occurred. There is also a notation of the fact that personal problems were raised during ward conference. No opinion is expressed. Only the facts are presented.

A note similar to the second one can be useful in presenting information about Miss McNeilly's performance. However, an isolated note of this type would hardly be meaningful. It could be used only if there were other notations about Miss McNeilly's behavior in a ward conference. One of the main problems with anecdotal notes is that they tend to be isolated fragments and often present one-time behaviors. Before it is possible to arrive at an objective evaluation of behavior, it is necessary to have information over a period of time based on observation of the performance of the individual with respect to a specific activity, or group of activities.

Consider another example of an anecdotal note:

Miss McNeilly lacks the ability to relate to patients. She always gets upset about doing personal things for patients. The patients don't like her.

This is another very subjective anecdotal note. No facts are presented to substantiate the statement that patients do not like Miss McNeilly. There is no indication of the time the behavior took place, or the particular situation involved.

In order to be useful, the note should contain information along the following lines:

On Jan. 8 Miss McNeilly waited at the door of Ward B for two or three minutes before entering. She said she was "trying to get up courage to face the patients." She said she "hates" to change dressings, particularly for men.

The patient near the window in Ward B complained that Miss McNeilly had made an unpleasant comment to him when she changed his dressing. She compared him unfavorably to her father. The patient said he felt depressed after Miss McNeilly's comments.

From this statement it is possible to derive a number of facts about Miss McNeilly's performance. The date is recorded. There is a record of the fact that she had difficulty approaching the patients in Ward B. There is a record of a statement of dislike for changing dressings. This is evidence of an unfavorable attitude about performing certain nursing functions. The fact that she caused the patient near the window to feel uncomfortable by her remarks is another act of undesirable performance. No opinions have been given, just statements about Miss McNeilly's behavior.

When anecdotal notes are written with due regard for accuracy of the facts, they can be extremely useful. In many ways they are superior to checklists or rating scales because observers are not forced into a rigid structure in describing behavior. However, it is the very latitude of anecdotal notes that often leads to difficulty. A common problem is the tendency to weigh personality factors too heavily in reporting behaviors. Often personal conflicts between student and instructor are evident in the manner in which anecdotal notes are written. Some observers find it difficult to be objective. Due to limitations of this type, anecdotal notes at times can be only marginally effective.

Perhaps the greatest difficulty in the use of anecdotal notes is the matter of developing some relationships among the various notations on a student's record. Before it is possible to get any impressions of the over-all behavior of the student in a given period of time, it is necessary to organize the anecdotal notes into some kind of framework. Often the notes bear little or no relationship to one another and for this reason it is difficult to use them. The burden of organizing the notes falls on the observer or on the person who is attempting to interpret the meaning of the notes in relation to the behavior of the student.

The Performance Record of Critical Incidents

An adaptation of the use of anecdotal notes that is considerably more objective is the performance record based on a collection of critical incidents of behavior. The details of this kind of information were presented in Chapter 2. In this section we will describe the use of critical incidents in an organized framework for use in presenting facts about performance.

Observers are asked to record specific critical incidents of effective or ineffective behavior. Each observer is briefed in advance about the definition of an incident and what kinds of behavior constitute critical incidents. In addition the observer has a list of behaviors divided into major and minor areas. This list helps to record incidents of behavior in a systematic way so that items describing similar types of behavior are grouped together. There is space on the form for a date, a classification of the item of behavior, and a brief notation of the facts about the situation.

There are always two sides to the performance record—one for recording effective performance and the other for ineffective performance. When behaviors are recorded on this type of record, they present trends of behavior that may be significant for student development. The performance record covers a specific period of time in the student's educational experience. For this reason it is possible to regard the incidents of behavior in direct relation to a point in time when specific behaviors occur.

Some of the advantages of recording critical incidents of performance on a systematic record are as follows:

1. The record is dated.
2. The notations contain no opinion or judgments.
3. The incidents present only the facts of performance.
4. The incidents can be recorded in an organized and systematic manner.
5. The organization of the record permits the information to be used to interpret trends of behavior.

An example of a performance record that was developed specifically for the purpose of recording observations of the performance of students and nursing practitioners is presented in the chapter on the Clinical Experience Record (Chapter 9).

INTERPRETING RESULTS OF EVALUATION

Scores on tests, or information about ratings and rankings, can be meaningful only if they are interpreted correctly and used constructively. Isolated scores on single tests should not be used as the basis for evaluating student performance. Evaluation should be based on the results of a number of tests and on several other factors. Micheels and Karnes suggest:

> For the course in which direct subject-matter objectives center in the development of manipulative skills as well as understandings, the results to be considered might include:
>
> 1. Scores on quizzes and short written tests
> 2. Scores on performance tests
> 3. Scores on comprehensive tests and term or final examinations
> 4. Data pertaining to daily performance in
>   a. classroom activities
>   b. on the unit
>   c. in the laboratory
> 5. Data recorded on certain observation checklists, progress charts (or on performance records)
> 6. Marks on completed projects
> 7. Marks on written assignments, special reports, etc.*

Judgments as to the assignment of relative weights or values for each of these factors should not be the responsibility of one person alone. Committees of faculty members should make decisions about the relative weights to assign each of the factors involved in reaching an over-all

* Micheels and Karnes, *op. cit.*, p. 417.

evaluation of performance. Micheels and Karnes suggest the following criteria:

1. Objective measures should receive greater weight than subjective ones.
2. Term, final, or comprehensive types of examinations should receive greater weight than short quizzes.
3. Cooperative projects or assignments should not receive too much weight because it is always difficult to determine the extent of the participation of each person and the amount of assistance they might have obtained from outside sources.
4. Time can be used as the basis for assigning weight to the acquisition of certain kinds of manipulative skills.
5. No one measure should constitute the basis for failure, with the possible exception of the final examination which covers the work of the entire semester. This final examination should only be accorded full weight for the pass-fail decision if it is a fully validated examination.*

These criteria were presented for programs in general education. They could readily be adapted for use in making evaluations of the performance of students in schools of nursing.

COMMUNICATION OF RESULTS TO STUDENTS

The interpretation of test scores is important from the standpoint of teaching, but it is equally important from the standpoint of the student. The instructor should use test results for the purpose of communicating valuable information to the student about the quality of her performance in relation to the content of the test and what implications these results may have.

For this reason, no instructor should present scores or grades on a test to students in the form of the score or grade alone. Students should be told the range of scores made by the class so that they are able to judge their standing in relation to others in the class. If grades are given on the test rather than percentile scores or raw scores, the grades should be presented together with information about the level of performance the grade includes. A grade of "C" tells a student that her performance was about midway in relation to the class. It does not tell her whether this was close to a "B" or close to a "D" or whether the performance was average or just fair. Scores or grades alone do not offer the student any basis on which to identify areas for improvement. No student can judge from a mere score which questions she answered correctly or which she answered incorrectly unless the instructor takes the time to go over the test pointing

* Micheels and Karnes, loc. cit.

out these facts. Tests should not only be used to test, they should also be used to teach.

Communication of results is also important when observers make records of the behaviors they observe. It is not sufficient for a student to know that she ranked eighth in a class of 22 in a performance test on preparing a patient for major surgery. The students should know in advance, during the time the learning experiences in this area are being presented, just what is regarded as an acceptable standard of behavior. In this way, assuming these same behaviors have been used as a checklist for observing performance, the student will have some basis on which to understand the meaning of the ranking. However, merely telling the student her rank in relation to the class is not sufficient. The student should be told about performance in behavioral terms so that she has a basis on which to make decisions about review and improvement of performance.

The most important function of evaluation is to provide the basis for guiding student progress. Mere letter grades, percentiles, or rankings do not provide any basis for scheduling remedial measures. Generalizations can mislead students. The student should be provided with the technical interpretation of her scores, with information about the score in relation to the performance of others in the class, and most importantly, with information about how to improve her performance. Teacher and student should work together to make the outcomes of evaluation worthwhile in terms of opportunities for professional growth and development.

Bibliography

Allport, George W. "The Use of Personal Documents in Psychological Science," *Social Science Research*, Monograph No. 49:12, 1942.

Anastasi, Anne. *Psychological Testing*, 2nd ed., The Macmillan Company, New York, 1961.

Cardew, Emily C. *Study Guide for Clinical Nursing*, rev. ed., J.B. Lippincott Company, Philadelphia, 1961.

Cronbach, Lee J. *Educational Psychology*, Harcourt, Brace and Company, Inc. New York, 1954.

Engelhart, Max D. "Improving Classroom Testing," *What Research Says to the Teacher*, No. 31, Department of Classroom Teachers, American Educational Research Association of the National Education Association, Washington, D.C., December, 1964.

Flanagan, John C. *The Clinical Experience Record Form*, Psychometric Techniques Associates, Pittsburgh, 1960.

Flanagan, John C., Marchese, Angeline C., Tuska, Shirley A., and Fivars, Grace. *Instructor's Manual for the Clinical Experience Record for Nursing Students*, Psychometric Techniques Associates, Pittsburgh, 1960.

Furst, Edward J. *Constructing Evaluation Instruments*, Longmans, Green & Company, Inc., New York, 1958.

Gorham, William A., Lichtenstein, Stanley, and Marchese, Angeline C. *Specific Nursing Behaviors Related to Patient Care and Improvement: Measuring Nursing Performance*, American Institutes for Research, Washington, D.C., May, 1959 (AIR-B-24-59-FR-204).

Gorham, William A. and staff. "Staff Nursing Behaviors Contributing to Patient Care and Improvement," *Nursing Research*, 11:68-79, 1962.

Micheels, William J., and Karnes, M. Ray. *Measuring Educational Achievement*, McGraw-Hill Series in Education, New York, 1950.

Rothney, J. W. M. "Evaluating and Reporting Pupil Progress," *What Research Says to the Teacher*, No. 7, Department of Classroom Teachers, American Educational Research Association of the National Education Association, Washington, D.C., March, 1955.

Sims, Verner M. "The Essay Examination Is a Projective Technique," *Educational and Psychological Measurement*, 8:15-31, (Jan.) 1948.

Spaulding, Geraldine. "Memo on Item Writing," and Appendix to Memo, unpublished document prepared for use by the staff of the American Institutes for Research, Pittsburgh, 1950.

Thorndike, Robert L., and Hagen, Elizabeth. *Measurement and Evaluation in Psychology and Education*, John Wiley & Sons, Inc., New York, 1961.

Wrightstone, J. Wayne, Justman, J., and Robbins, I. *Evaluation in Modern Education*, American Book Company, New York, 1956.

Selected References

American Institutes for Research. "Situational Tests of Leadership," *Research Note*, No. 8, American Institutes for Research, Pittsburgh, 1953.

American Institutes for Research. "Situational Tests for Evaluating Supervisory Skill," *Research Note*, No. 14, American Institutes for Research, Pittsburgh, 1957.

Flanagan, John C. "The Use of Comprehensive Rationales," *Educational and Psychological Measurement*, 11:151-55, 1951.

Flanagan, John C., *et al.* "Situational Performance Tests: A Symposium," *Personnel Psychology*, 7:461-97, 1954.

Flanagan, John C., and Burns, Robert K. "The Employee Performance Record: A New Appraisal and Development Tool," *Harvard Business Review*, 33: 95-102, 1955.

Flitter, Hessel. "Achievement Test in the Natural Sciences in Nursing," *Nursing Outlook*, 7:410-13, (July) 1959.

Glaser, Robert, Schwarz, Paul A., and Flanagan, John C. *Development of Interview and Performance Tests for the Selection of Wage Board Supervisers*, The Adjutant General's Office, Personnel Research Branch, Washington, D.C., Technical Research Note 53, 1956.

Holton, Gerald, "Testing and Self-Discovery," *University College Quarterly*, November, 1963.

Lindquist, E. F. *Educational Measurement*, American Council on Education, Washington, D.C. 1951. (Especially Chapter 7, "Writing the Test Item," by Robert L. Ebel.)

McLaughlin, Kenneth F. *Interpretation of Test Results*, U.S. Office of Education, Department of Health, Education, and Welfare, Washington, D.C., 1964.

National League for Nursing. "The Use of Tests in Schools of Nursing," *The Construction and Use of Teacher-Made Tests*, Pamphlet No. 5, The League, New York, 1957.

Weislogel, Mary H. *Development of a Test for Selecting Research Personnel,* American Institutes for Research, Pittsburgh, 1950 (AIR-A18-50-FR-12).

Wood, Dorothy Adkins. *Test Construction, Development, and Interpretation of Achievement Tests,* Charles E. Merrill Company, Columbus, 1960.

Critical Incident

The clinical instructor reviewed the student's strengths and weaknesses on her performance record (the Clinical Experience Record) at the completion of the course and experience in obstetric nursing.

The student stated she had enjoyed this experience very much. She had written down her weaknesses in advance of the conference. During the conference she asked the instructor to assist her in planning for improvement of these weaknesses since she would like to make obstetrics her area of specialization after graduation.

This is an effective incident in seeking additional opportunities for learning and asking for guidance when needed. The student recognized the value in planning for progress.

Chapter 9
Evaluation in
Terms of
Performance

Will the critical incident technique lend itself to evaluation of nursing behavior? Can it be used to evaluate on-the-job behavior? Where are incidents recorded? How are the records kept?

USING CRITICAL INCIDENTS
TO EVALUATE PERFORMANCE

A collection of critical incidents made on the basis of day-to-day observation of the performance of students, general practitioners, and others engaged in providing nursing functions can provide important insights into on-the-job behavior. Flanagan, Marchese, Tuska and Fivars did a study to determine whether critical incidents could be used to evaluate nursing performance.* More than 2000 incidents were collected in ten Pittsburgh area hospitals from schools of nursing enrolling from 75 to 400 students. The data collected included anecdotal notes and written incidents reported by instructors, supervisors, head nurses, general duty nurses, patients, and doctors. Even the students participated by writing incidents they had observed on one another. The data were sorted and analyzed on the basis of behaviors that were critical to the performance of nursing functions. A preliminary form was developed which included 18 major areas of behavior. Following the tryout, the procedures were modified and revised on the basis of the suggestions of the instructors and head nurses who participated in the study.

A new evaluation form was developed—a performance record to be used in evaluating nursing behavior.†

* John C. Flanagan, Angeline C. Marchese, Shirley A. Tuska, and Grace Fivars. *Instructor's Manual for the Clinical Experience Record for Nursing Students*, Psychometric Techniques Associates, Pittsburgh, 1960.

† Flanagan *et al., loc. cit.* John C. Flanagan. *The Clinical Experience Record for Nursing Students*, Psychometric Techniques Associates, Pittsburgh, 1960.

WHAT IS A
PERFORMANCE RECORD?

The *performance record* is a two-page form for recording critical incidents. One side is blue for recording effective incidents; the other is red to include notations of ineffective incidents. The form is divided into sections with captions of behaviors critical to nursing.

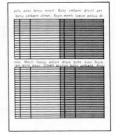

Front of Form   Double Spread Shows   Back of Form
                         12 Areas of Behavior

Figure 9   Miniature view of the *Clinical Experience Record.*

A look at the sample performance record will show the format used for the *Clinical Experience Record for Nursing Students:* An evaluation tool for recording critical incidents of nursing behavior. This was the final form developed by Flanagan *et al.,* on the basis of the project conducted in Pittsburgh.

The form contains a list of 12 major areas of behavior:

1. Planning, organizing, and adapting nursing care
2. Checking
3. Meeting the patient's adjustment and emotional needs
4. Meeting the patient's physical and medical needs
5. Applying scientific principles to nursing care
6. Observing, reporting, and charting
7. Adaptability to new or stressful situations
8. Relations with co-workers, physicians, and visitors
9. Judgment regarding professional values
10. Use of learning opportunities
11. Acceptance of nursing service responsibility
12. Personal appearance

Under each of these major areas are subheadings of behaviors appropriate to the general category. Spaces are provided for recording the date, the item number of the behavior, and a brief description of what happened. This is a record of the facts about performance, with a list of critical incidents identifying effective and ineffective behaviors.

Name _____ Class _____ Department or clinical area _____

<u>Memoranda on Progress</u>

For period beginning _____ to _____

Summary of incidents

Headings	1	2	3	4	5	6	7	8	9	10	11	12
Number of effective incidents												
Number of ineffective incidents												

Summary notes on . . .

Student's strong points: _____

_____
_____
_____
_____

Specific actions taken by student and supervisor: _____

_____
_____
_____
_____

Needs for improvement; sources of problems: _____

_____
_____
_____
_____

Results: Actions found to be effective or ineffective: _____

_____
_____
_____
_____

Further comments and suggestions for planning improvement or remedial actions: _____

_____
_____
_____
_____

Student's comments: _____

_____
_____
_____
_____

Instructor's Signature _____

Student's Signature _____

Date _____

Date _____

Figure 10 *The Clinical Experience Record.* (© Copyright 1960 by John C. Flanagan. Reproduced by permission.)

150

Behaviors to Be Encouraged

1. Planning, organizing, and adapting nursing care

   A. Organized nursing care plan or equipment efficiently.
   B. Anticipated needs of others.
   C. Adapted nursing care plan to overcome difficulties.
   D. Adapted nursing care procedures to patient's needs.
   E. Used adequate substitute equipment when necessary.
   F. Devised or suggested new technique for welfare of patient or for ward efficiency.

Date	Item	What Happened

2. Checking

   A. Checked Kardex frequently for new orders.
   B. Made special checks in medication procedure.
   C. Checked to see that laboratory orders were carried out.
   D. Noted inconsistency in medication, treatment, diet order.
   E. Checked equipment and supplies for shortage or defects.
   F. Made special checks on signs and condition of patient.

Date	Item	What Happened

3. Meeting the patient's adjustment and emotional needs

   A. Was reassuring, kind, and considerate to patient.
   B. Made arrangements for recreational or diversional therapy.
   C. Noted social service, home nursing, spiritual, other needs.
   D. Adapted explanation of teaching to patient's understanding.
   E. Effectively taught patient health principles or home care.

Date	Item	What Happened

Student's Name

Behaviors Needing Improvement

1. Planning, organizing, and adapting nursing care
   a. Failed to organize nursing care for maximum patient benefit.
   b. Failed to collect all equipment necessary for patient care.
   c. Took unwise shortcuts in giving nursing care.
   d. Failed to adapt procedure to situation.
   e. Used inadequate or improper substitute equipment.

Date	Item	What Happened

2. Checking
   a. Failed to check Kardex in administering medication, treatment.
   b. Did not check cards, labels, or names in medication procedure.
   c. Failed to see that laboratory orders were carried out.
   d. Did not question inconsistent medication, treatment, diet order.
   e. Failed to check requisition, equipment, or supplies.
   f. Neglected to check patient's condition.

Date	Item	What Happened

3. Meeting the patient's adjustment and emotional needs
   a. Refused request, was unkind, tactless, or indifferent.
   b. Did not provide recreational or diversional activity.
   c. Failed to recognize social service, spiritual, other needs.
   d. Did not explain or reassure patient about test, treatment, or policy; or misinformed patient.

Date	Item	What Happened

Behaviors to Be Encouraged

4. Meeting the patient's physical and medical needs
   A. Carried out medical order or nursing care procedure correctly despite difficulties.
   B. Made use of comfort or nursing care measures until medical orders could be obtained.
   C. Made environmental changes for patient's welfare or safety.
   D. Was very skillful or gentle in giving nursing care.

Date	Item	What Happened

5. Applying scientific principles to nursing care
   A. Exhibited understanding of advanced nursing principles.
   B. Questioned situation which violated underlying principles.

Date	Item	What Happened

6. Observing, reporting, and charting
   A. Noticed and reported special physical, emotional, or social need of patient.
   B. Immediately reported new symptoms or significant change.
   C. Reported why medication or treatment could not be given.
   D. Reported significant facts to relief nurse.
   E. Wrote excellent nurse's notes.

Date	Item	What Happened

Behaviors Needing Improvement

4. Meeting the patient's physical and medical needs
   a. Made error in giving medication, treatment, or other nursing care.
   b. Ignored or failed to carry out orders.
   c. Overlooked need for improvement or safety in environment.
   d. Caused patient discomfort due to lack of skill, awkwardness.
   e. Did not prepare patient properly for test, treatment, procedure.

Date	Item	What Happened

5. Applying scientific principles to nursing care

   a. Did not know vital theory or principles of nursing care.

   b. Ignored or failed to apply scientific principles.

Date	Item	What Happened

6. Observing, reporting, and charting
   a. Failed to notice need for special patient care.
   b. Failed to report significant facts about patient's condition.
   c. Failed to report off duty or to report unfinished patient care.
   d. Failed to chart treatment, observations, or nursing care.
   e. Charted or transcribed incorrectly or incompletely.

Date	Item	What Happened

154

Behaviors to Be Encouraged

7. Adaptability to new or stressful situations

    A. Required minimum guidance in adjusting to new situation.
    B. Learned new procedure or skill quickly.
    C. Carried out nursing care calmly and efficiently under stress.
    D. Took immediate and appropriate action in an emergency.

Date	Item	What Happened

8. Relations with co-workers, physicians, and visitors

    A. Was tactful in handling difficult situation.

    B. Was cooperative with co-workers, physicians, other personnel.

    C. Assisted in instruction and supervision of auxiliary personnel.

Date	Item	What Happened

9. Judgment regarding professional values

    A. Called attention to own error which was otherwise unnoticed.
    B. Reported situation accurately despite reflection on self.
    C. Kept information confidential despite pressure to divulge it.
    D. Maintained ethical standards in a difficult situation.

Date	Item	What Happened

Behaviors Needing Improvement

7. Adaptability to new or stressful situations

    a. Adjusted slowly or required excessive guidance.
    b. Was very slow in developing manual skill in new technique.
    c. Became tense, upset, or disorganized under stress.
    d. Caused delay or took inappropriate action in an emergency.

Date	Item	What Happened

8. Relations with co-workers, physicians, and visitors

    a. Was tactless or rude to visitor or hospital personnel.
    b. Failed to cooperate with co-workers or others.
    c. Did not use opportunity for teaching auxiliary personnel.
    d. Interfered with instruction, supervision, or work of others.

Date	Item	What Happened

9. Judgment regarding professional values

    a. Tried to cover up or denied obvious errors.
    b. Made exaggerated statements about nursing care given.
    c. Used poor judgment about releasing confidential information.
    d. Used questionable judgment in ethical matter.

Date	Item	What Happened

156

Behaviors to Be Encouraged

10. Use of learning opportunities
    A. Made significant contribution to ward conference.
    B. Expended extra effort to follow through on patient care.
    C. Asked to observe or learn a new procedure.
    D. Accepted suggestions and criticism graciously.
    E. Asked for supervision or guidance when needed.

Date	Item	What Happened

11. Acceptance of nursing service responsibility
    A. Voluntarily assumed extra duties within limits of responsibility.
    B. Willingly cooperated with assignment or schedule change.
    C. Followed established policy or procedure despite difficulties.
    D. Assumed leadership or management responsibilities as needed.
    E. Took care to conserve supplies and equipment.

Date	Item	What Happened

12. Personal appearance
    A. Made change in grooming which improved personal appearance.

Date	Item	What Happened

Behaviors Needing Improvement

10. <u>Use of learning opportunities</u>
    a. Did not participate in or prepare for ward conference.
    b. Failed to keep clinical records up to date.
    c. Failed to take advantage of opportunity to learn.
    d. Was defensive, indignant, or indifferent about criticism.
    e. Failed to ask for guidance or went to improper authority.

Date	Item	What Happened

11. <u>Acceptance of nursing service responsibility</u>
    a. Ignored or refused task beyond assignment or responsibilities.
    b. Was uncooperative in schedule or assignment change.
    c. Deviated from established policy or procedure.
    d. Arrived on department unnecessarily late.
    e. Wasted, destroyed, or damaged supplies or equipment.

Date	Item	What Happened

12. <u>Personal appearance</u>
    a. Failed to wear uniform as required.
    b. Appeared untidy, not well groomed.

Date	Item	What Happened

Additional Notes on Clinical Experience Record Incidents

Enter below any incidents for which there is insufficient space on the preceding pages. Refer to date and item number.

Behaviors to Be Encouraged.   Behaviors Needing Improvement

Date	Heading and Item	What Happened	Date	Heading and Item	What Happened

Enter below incidents which cannot be classified under the headings on the preceding pages. Describe these incidents in detail, so that someone who did not actually observe the incident will be able to tell what happened.

Date		What Happened	Date		What Happened

LEARNING PERFORMANCE
RECORD PROCEDURES

Learning to Think in Terms of Critical Incidents

Observation of critical incidents can become an implicit part of every-day activities. When you learn to think in terms of incidents that are critical, irrelevant issues are eliminated, only important facts remain. These are the facts that you will record on the *Clinical Experience Record*.

Incidents happen all the time, in every nursing situation. But all incidents are not critical. A critical incident is one that makes a significant difference in the outcome of an activity. It may be the positive factor that contributes toward the success of the behavior, or it may be the negative factor that interferes with the completion of the assignment. Instructors should have no difficulty in recognizing critical incidents if they use the 12 major areas of behavior as a guide to thinking. Once you learn to think in these terms, it is not difficult to determine whether an incident is effective or ineffective, and what effect it has on the outcome of the activity you observe.

The following suggestions should guide you in learning to think in terms of critical incidents:

1. Study the aim of the activity. Make a list of the behaviors that are important. (See list of expected behaviors in Appendix II.)
2. Establish minimum standards for acceptable performance in each clinical area. (These should be based on course objectives.)
3. Learn to eliminate halo effects, personal feelings, and biases.
4. Learn to concentrate on incidents that are significant. Ask the question: Did this make an important difference in the outcome of the assignment?
5. Learn to determine priorities when several things occur simultaneously. Identify significant behaviors of both types when events occur in rapid succession.
6. Observe the total situation, not isolated aspects of it.
7. Learn to evaluate the whole student, not just fragments of her behavior.
8. Observe incidents continuously as you teach and as students perform.
9. Record incidents daily. This reduces a tendency to forget. Memory often distorts the facts when you wait until the end of the week to record incidents. Recording takes only a few minutes. Do it each day.
10. Record only the facts. No opinions, judgments, or conclusions need be included—just the facts.

11. Learn to observe in relation to the level at which the student is performing. You cannot expect a first-level student to display the competence of a second-level student. Advanced students should be expected to perform at a level superior to intermediate students. Practitioners should maintain a level of performance consistent with professional standards.

12. Discuss an incident as soon as possible after it occurs. Take the time to talk with the nurse you have observed and to tell her what you observed that was effective or ineffective. The critical incident technique involves no secrecy; both observers and participants share in the responsibility of writing the record. For this reason, when an incident is observed, it should be brought to the nurse's attention as soon as possible after she leaves the patient.

Learning to Observe Critical Incidents

Experience has indicated that observers are most successful when they have a good working knowledge of the activity they are to observe. In nursing the observer is either an instructor, a head nurse, or someone responsible for general supervision of nursing activities. Each person should have a thorough knowledge of the behaviors important to success in the activity being observed. Instructors should develop lists of behaviors for each clinical area. These can be reviewed with the students so that they know what is expected of them in each area. Samples of lists of expected behaviors are included in Appendix II.

Learning experiences should include a review of the behaviors that are important to successful performance for each type of nursing care. When both instructors and students are familiar with the list of behaviors, evaluation can proceed more systematically. Instructors have a good basis on which to observe critical incidents, and students are well aware of the aspects of their behavior that are important in carrying out their assignments.

Using a list of expected behaviors, observers should learn to note (for an assignment involving a procedure):

1. Preparation to give nursing care
   a. The development of a nursing care plan
   b. The preparation of materials, supplies, and equipment required
2. Preparation of the patient for the procedure
   a. The preliminary discussion with the patient to advise him of tests to be taken, or procedures to be carried out
   b. The physical preparation of the patient
3. Sequencing of steps in the appropriate order to accomplish the procedure efficiently
4. Manner in which procedure is carried out
   a. Observation of sterile techniques

b. Best use of equipment

c. Consideration for the comfort of the patient

5. Follow-up after procedure is completed

a. Consideration of the comfort of the patient

b. Recording nurse's notes

c. Disposal of waste matter

d. Analysis of specimen if necessary, making appropriate tests

e. Reporting of findings to appropriate persons as necessary

Each clinical area of nursing, of course, will have its own set of behaviors to be observed and its own criteria for successful completion of an assignment. Each instructor should impress her students with the importance of learning to do procedures in the manner described in the nursing procedure book or according to established criteria. Acceptable standards are the only standards to consider. Students will eventually be practitioners, and it will be their obligation to maintain professional standards. If learning experiences emphasize high standards, performance should be of equal quality.

What Is Reasonable Behavior?

Fixed procedures are relatively easy to observe since there are step-by-step sequences to be carried out to accomplish the assignment. In observing procedures it should not be too difficult to identify omissions and oversights, or to decide when a behavior is insufficient or inadequate.

However, many aspects in nursing require behavior that is somewhat different. Nursing requires the application of communication techniques, interpersonal relationships, awareness of signs and symptoms, ability to maintain composure in a trying situation, heavy schedules, sharing responsibility, judgment, and a gentle manner. Instructors and others who are charged with the assignment of observing nursing behavior must keep all these requirements in mind as they record critical incidents. Each behavior is important to success in nursing; combinations of several may occur in various situations. Emergencies occur constantly, and nurses should be able to cope with them. When emergencies develop, it is often necessary to modify procedures or patient care accordingly. Observers should be alert to the manner in which this is done and should be careful not to overemphasize routine approaches when some modification is necessary. On the other hand, observers should use the established standards as a basis for making judgments about the critical aspects of behavior. Carelessness, lack of understanding, or intolerant behavior are often noticeable in day-to-day routine activities. An instructor should be cautious about permitting the standard of performance to drop below the level of acceptability. Excellence in nursing can be achieved only if instructors learn to identify behaviors that are reasonable to expect of students as they carry out their assignments, and to reinforce a high standard of acceptability.

For example, if a second-year or intermediate student is observed making a patient's bed with the side rails up, this should be recognized immediately as an ineffective incident for this student at her particular level. An intermediate student should be well aware of the need for using good body mechanics in giving patient care.

To take another example, if a beginning student were assigned the care of a patient with a communicable disease, and she voluntarily used an isolation bag for bed linens, this would be an effective incident. For a beginning student, this would be evidence of the use of good judgment in applying scientific principles regarding infection.

Often assignments are complex, and the expected behaviors are not always clear-cut or easy to identify. Observers should use lists of expected behaviors to determine what is reasonable behavior for the student at her level of education. Using this as a basis, observation should proceed in reference to the behavior of the student. If the behavior is outstanding, the student should be commended and encouraged. If the behavior is below the accepted standard, the student should be told what she did that was ineffective and how she should go about improving her behavior.

What About Average Performance?

In every class and in every working situation there are people who tend to do just what is expected, no more and no less. Their performance would be regarded as average. These are the "C" students in the classroom situation, the "average" nurses in the employment situation. How does an observer handle this type of performance?

No school of nursing should be satisfied to produce "just average" nurses. Every instructor should strive to stimulate her students to the point that they are not satisfied just to "get by" or "just pass" in a course. Nursing is a highly demanding profession; there is little room for apathy. The very nature of nursing is challenging; each patient contact presents a new set of problems, and these should be handled with care and a sincere effort to make the patient comfortable. Try to encourage the student to be enthusiastic about her profession and to undertake each new assignment with a determination to provide a high quality of patient care.

Motivation is a vital factor. If an instructor can succeed in motivating her students toward higher achievement in nursing, she may be able to instill in them the habit of working toward higher goals. If you have some of the so-called "average" students with whom you can find no fault, but who never do anything outstanding, try to present these students with special problems to challenge their imaginations. Many an instructor will be surprised to find that an erstwhile average student can move quickly to avert an emergency when finally put in the position of responsibility. If necessary, create an "emergency" problem and place the average student in charge of handling the difficulty. If she succeeds, you may find you no longer have just an "average" student. If, on the other hand, she fails to cope with the stressful situation, you have a basis on which to try to overcome the student's weaknesses. It is often possible to awaken the interest of students by giving them additional assignments of the type that cannot be handled in the average way.

HOW TO RECORD
A CRITICAL INCIDENT

Once you learn to observe critical incidents and to determine what is reasonable behavior, it should be easy to learn how to keep the record. Incidents should be recorded every day as soon as possible after they occur. These simple steps should help in keeping the record:

1. Determine whether the incident you observed is critical.
2. Was it effective or ineffective?
3. How would you classify the behavior?
   a. Review the 12 major areas of behavior on the Clinical Experience Record form. Decide which is appropriate for the behavior you observed.
   b. Read through the subcategories to identify the one that is most descriptive of the behavior you observed.
   c. Note the number of the main heading and the letter designation of the subheading.
4. Record the incident
   a. You may prefer to use incident slips to make your first record of an incident. These are convenient 3 × 5 slips on which you can write out the details of an incident and make a preliminary classification. (See sample form in Fig. 12.)
   b. Write the date, using number designations, e.g., 7/26 represents July 26.
   c. Write the number of the major heading and the letter of the subheading, e.g., 4C.

4. Meeting the patient's physical and medical needs

   A. Carried out medical order or nursing care procedure correctly despite difficulties.
   B. Made use of comfort or nursing care measures until medical orders could be obtained.
   C. Made environmental changes for patient's welfare or safety.
   D. Was very skillful or gentle in giving nursing care.

7/26	C	*Removed casters from bed*

5. Applying scientific principles to nursing care

   A. Exhibited understanding of advanced nursing principles.

Figure 11 Example of an incident recorded on the *Clinical Experience Record.*

FOR EFFECTIVE INCIDENTS

Student's
Name _____   Observed
                                by _____   Date _____

Item	Behavior Category	Describe exactly what happened.
_____	1. Planning, org. & adapting nursing care.	
_____	2. Checking.	
_____	3. Meeting patient's adj. & emotional needs.	
_____	4. Meeting patient's phys. & medical needs.	
_____	5. Applying scientific principles.	
_____	6. Observing, reporting, and charting.	
_____	7. Adaptability to new/stressful situations.	
_____	8. Rel. with co-workers, physicians, visitors.	
_____	9. Judgment regarding professional values.	
_____ 10.	Use of learning opportunities.	
_____ 11.	Accept. of nursing service responsibility.	
_____ 12.	Personal appearance.	

What did student do that was effective/ineffective?

Figure 12A   Incident form for recording an *effective* critical incident.

This indicates an incident under heading 4—*Meeting the patient's physical and medical needs,* and subheading C—*Made environmental changes for patient's welfare or safety.*

d. Describe what happened. Use as few words as possible to indicate the action observed. For example, "removed casters from bed" would be sufficient to inform the reader that the nurse had removed the casters from the bed to provide a safer environment for the patient.

The finished incident on the record is shown in Figure 11.

If the incident slip was used first, more detail would be written to indicate the fact that the patient was in a cast. At the end of the week, this slip would be used to transfer the incident to the performance record form, and the item would be written for the record.

FOR INEFFECTIVE INCIDENTS

Student's
Name _____

Observed
by _____   Date _____

Item	Behavior Category	Describe exactly what happened.
_____	1. Planning, org. & adapting nursing care.	
_____	2. Checking.	
_____	3. Meeting patient's adj. & emotional needs.	
_____	4. Meeting patient's phys. & medical needs.	
_____	5. Applying scientific principles.	
_____	6. Observing, reporting, and charting.	
_____	7. Adaptability to new/stressful situations.	
_____	8. Rel. with co-workers, physicians, visitors.	
_____	9. Judgment regarding professional values.	
_____	10. Use of learning opportunities.	
_____	11. Accept. of nursing service responsibility.	
_____	12. Personal appearance.	

What did student do that was effective/ineffective?

Figure 12B   Incident form for recording an *ineffective* critical incident.

Can You Record These Incidents?

Incident 1

A patient was recovering from abdominal surgery and needed continuous gastric suction. Miss Thomas, an advanced student, charted no drainage for the 7:00 to 3:00 tour. She immediately investigated the equipment and noted that it was defective. She replaced it and then checked several times to make certain the drainage was taking place.

1. Is this an incident?
2. Is it critical?
3. Is it effective or ineffective?
4. How would you classify it on the record?
5. How would you describe what happened?

ANSWERS

1. Yes, it is an incident.
2. It is critical.
3. It is effective.
4. The classification would be—
   2 Checking
      F Made special checks on signs and conditions of patient.

In patient care the important consideration is the patient's condition. In this instance the nurse noted the lack of drainage where drainage was important to patient welfare. She then inspected the equipment and found it was defective. She replaced it, thereby providing a situation for greater patient comfort.

5. This should be written as follows:
   Replaced faulty equipment.
   or
   Checked drainage flow, equipment.

Each instructor will have her own method for recording in short descriptive terms the incidents that occur. Try to use words that will convey as much information in as few words as possible.

In discussing this incident with the nurse it would be appropriate to commend her for her alertness in noting the defective equipment. The most important fact, however, is that she replaced the equipment and continued to check on the patient to make certain the equipment was functioning. Mention this and encourage the student to continue to behave in this manner.

Suppose this same situation had occurred and a beginning student had been involved. What would be the expected behavior in this case? First, a beginning student has less experience in handling problems of this type and may not have been taught how to replace gastric drainage equipment.

The beginning student should be expected to note important signs and symptoms, however. In this instance if she noted no drainage she should immediately have notified the appropriate person. If the student came to you, the instructor, and told you that the drainage equipment was not functioning, this would be an effective behavior for this student *at her level*. She could not reasonably be expected to replace or adjust the equipment because she has not had sufficient experience to be able to do this. The appropriate person should arrange to replace the equipment. If the student is still giving care to the same patient, she should be shown how the equipment is put into use so that when she checks on the patient's condition later, she will be able to tell whether the equipment is in good working order and still functioning.

If an advanced student had noted the defective equipment and had come to you to tell you about it, this would be an ineffective incident. At an advanced level the student should be familiar with the operation of drainage equipment, should know when it is defective, and should initiate steps to have it replaced or adjusted. She should not need to tell someone about the problem. She should be able to handle it herself.

On the following pages we have illustrated an incident in each of the major areas of behavior, one effective and one ineffective. There is a discussion of the incident, and the appropriate classification is indicated. Read through the incidents and note the way in which they are classified. Practice of this type should enable you to classify the incidents you observe in your daily teaching.

SAMPLE INCIDENTS AND THEIR CLASSIFICATION ON THE CLINICAL EXPERIENCE RECORD

The following are samples of incidents of behavior which have been classified on the basis of—

1. *Actual observation of the events surrounding the incident.*
2. *Consideration of the level of the student.*
3. *Relevance of the behavior to the general aim of the activity involved.*

Behavior Area 1
Planning, Organizing, and Adapting Nursing Care.

The main emphasis in this area is on skills in planning and organizing the nursing care plan and adapting that care or aspects of it to the patient's needs. It also involves transferring knowledge of certain principles of care from the classroom or laboratory situation to the bedside situation.

INCIDENT:

Miss Midway, an intermediate-level student, had difficulty in positioning a laminectomy patient on a bedpan. She immediately substituted a fracture pan for the patient's comfortable usage.

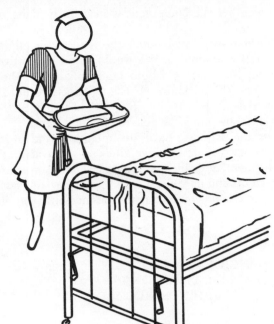

1. Planning, organizing, and adapting nursing care

    A. Organized nursing care plan or equipment efficiently.
    B. Anticipated needs of others.
    C. Adapted nursing care plan to overcome difficulties.
    D. Adapted nursing care procedures to patient's needs.
    E. Used adequate substitute equipment when necessary.
    F. Devised or suggested new technique for welfare of
       patient or for ward efficiency.

2/1	1D	*Substituted fracture pan*

Rationale for classification: This is a situation in which at first glance several of the behaviors listed might apply. For example: (1) The nurse used an adequate substitution for the regulation bedpan, thus a possible classification would be under E. (2) It might also appear appropriate to consider this a situation in which the nurse adapted the nursing care plan to overcome difficulties as in C. (3) However, the nurse's real concern was for the patient's comfort, thus the item that is the most appropriate would be 1D, "Adapted nursing care procedures to patient's needs."

INCIDENT:

Miss Older, an advanced-level student, during the process of performing a catheterization discovered she had neglected to place the lubricant on the sterile tray. She asked the nurse's aide to bring the lubricant to the patient's bedside.

This is an incident of ineffective behavior. The classification for this incident should not be difficult to find because item 1b, "Failed to collect all equipment necessary for patient care," is a clear description of exactly what happened.

1. Planning, organizing, and adapting nursing care
     a. Failed to organize nursing care for maximum patient benefit.
     b. Failed to collect all equipment necessary for patient care.
     c. Took unwise shortcuts in giving nursing care.
     d. Failed to adapt procedure to situation.
     e. Used inadequate or improper substitute equipment.

2/10	1 b	Forgot lubricant for cath. tray

Note, in recording incidents, it is appropriate to record only the month and day date. The year date should appear on the front of the folder, so it is not really necessary to repeat it on the inside chart. It is also suggested that the major behavior area be indicated by number and the subcategory by letter. Note that effective behaviors are indicated by upper-case letters, A, B, C, whereas ineffective behaviors are indicated by lower-case letters, a, b, c. In recording "what happened" it is suggested that the incident be described in concise terms. There is no need for paragraphs or sentences, just a few words should serve as a reminder of the incident. If the instructor feels a strong need to record more detail, an incident slip is available for this purpose. Some instructors prefer to fill out the incident slips first just to get the information down on paper. They then transfer the incident to the record. This plan works out very well, because many instructors prefer to carry just the small incident slips with them.

Behavior Area 2
Checking

An important activity for any nurse, regardless of her status as a student, a graduate, an instructor, a head nurse, or any other capacity in which she might give nursing care, is checking. All aspects of her work must be carefully checked. Because errors or omissions can have such serious implications for the patient, every nurse must make systematic checking an integral part of her pattern of behavior.

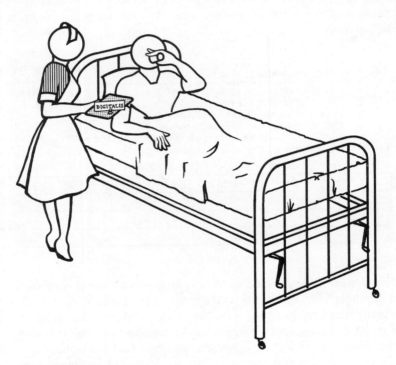

INCIDENT:

Miss Older, an advanced-level student, was assigned the responsibility for the nursing care of four medical patients. One was ambulatory; the other three were acutely ill and required constant attention. In her hurry to cover the assignment Miss Older did not check the pulse rate of one of her patients before administering digitalis.

2. Checking

    a. Failed to check Kardex in administering medication, treatment.
    b. Did not check cards, labels, or names in medication procedure.
    c. Failed to see that laboratory orders were carried out.
    d. Did not question inconsistent medication, treatment, diet order.
    e. Failed to check requisition, equipment, or supplies.
    f. Neglected to check patient's condition.

12/8	2f	gave digitalis, did not ck. pulse

Rationale for classification: In this incident, there is little problem about the important issue. A primary consideration is always the condition of the patient. The condition of the patient's pulse is of particular importance when there is an order for digitalis. Since the nurse failed to check the patient's pulse, this item would be classified as item 2f.

INCIDENT:

Miss Young, a first-level student, noted a discrepancy between the dosage of a drug on the Kardex and that on the medicine card. She checked the doctor's order and then notified the head nurse.

2. Checking

    A. Checked Kardex frequently for new orders.
    B. Made special checks in medication procedure.
    C. Checked to see that laboratory orders were carried out.
    D. Noted inconsistency in medication, treatment, diet order.
    E. Checked equipment and supplies for shortage or defects.
    F. Made special checks on signs and condition of patient.

2/16	2D	Discrepancy on med. card

In any situation where many people work together, there are possibilities that human errors will enter the situation. Sometimes there are transcription errors; at times numbers are transposed; there could possibly be an error in the selection of the appropriate chart on which to record information. It is hoped that the number of these errors would be kept to a minimum. However, there are still chances that such errors will occur. For this reason, it is important to check medication dosage figures. If there is a discrepancy, it could be a clerical error of transcription. Regardless of what the cause of the error might have been, the important thing at this student's level was to check with someone who could give her the correct information. In this case, the student checked with the head nurse. This was an effective behavior for a student at the first level. The appropriate classification for this behavior would be 2D.

Behavior Area 3
Meeting the Patient's Adjustment and Emotional Needs

The nurse must learn to know her patient and to recognize subtle, covert problems or needs. She should be able to understand and comfort the patient in a difficult situation. Patient needs differ. One may require firmness; another may need kindness and constant reassurance. The nurse must be prepared in this area to teach health habits, to be aware of the patient's total needs, to be familiar with sources of social, religious, or other aids, to be able to provide for recreational activity for the patient, and to be able to explain or discuss procedures with the patient in terms the patient is able to understand.

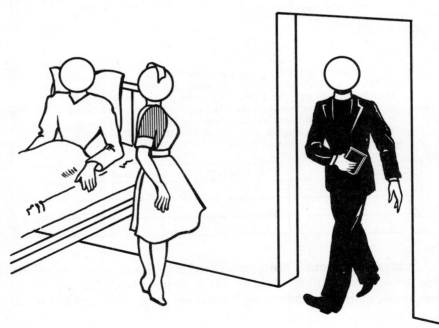

INCIDENT:

Miss Young, a first-level student, was giving care to a preoperative patient who asked several questions about the religious facilities of the hospital. She informed the patient the hospital had a chaplain service and arranged for a visit from the chaplain at the patient's request.

3. Meeting the patient's adjustment and emotional needs
   A. Was reassuring, kind, and considerate to patient.
   B. Made arrangements for recreational or diversional therapy.
   C. Noted social service, home nursing, spiritual, other needs.
   D. Adapted explanation of teaching to patient's understanding.
   E. Effectively taught patient health principles or home care.

3/2	3C	*Arr. for visit fr. Chaplain*

This type of incident should be easy to classify. The appropriate category would be 3C, "Noted social service, home nursing, *spiritual*, or other needs." The nurse should be able to guide the conversation so that the patient is led to express his wishes in a certain matter. For example, in this case the patient may simply have asked about religious facilities. It shouldn't be too difficult for the nurse to realize that the patient may be seeking spiritual comfort. In cases where the patient may not be so verbal, the nurse may need to use her judgment about leading the conversation to the next step, the matter of whether the patient would like to have more information or possibly a visit from the chaplain. A glance at the patient's background information will enable the nurse to make the decision about the appropriate chaplain to call.

INCIDENT:

Miss Midway, an intermediate-level student, was caring for an apprehensive preoperative patient who inquired if she knew the time (hour) his surgery was scheduled. She responded, "I do not know," and proceeded to make his bed.

The classification of this incident could be under item 3d, "Did not explain or reassure patient. . . ." However, a more appropriate classification in

3. Meeting the patient's adjustment and emotional needs

   a. Refused request, was unkind, tactless, or indifferent.
   b. Did not provide recreational or diversional activity.
   c. Failed to recognize social service, spiritual, other needs.
   d. Did not explain or reassure patient about test, treatment, or policy; or misinformed patient.

1/24	3a	Was indiff. to pt. inquiry

this case would be item 3a, "Refused request, was unkind, tactless, or indifferent." In this situation the nurse was both unkind and indifferent. Her short answer could indicate to a sensitive patient that she did not care. The fact that she went on with the bed-making without an effort to find out the answer to the patient's question was an indication of indifference. She could have mentioned to the patient that she would make an effort to find out about the time of surgery as soon as she finished making the bed. In this way, she would have been able to continue taking care of the immediate problem of making the patient's bed, but she also would have been giving the patient a form of assurance by indicating that she would attempt to find the answer to his question. The classification in this case would be 3a.

Behavior Area 4
Meeting the Patient's Physical and Medical Needs

Emphasis in this area is on the nurse's technical and fundamental skills. Providing for the physical and environmental needs of the patient involves the correct use of equipment, the ability to adjust or modify certain routines to cope with patient needs. A good basic knowledge of procedures, practice, and policy is required in this area, together with some ingenuity in being able to make minor environmental changes for patient safety.

INCIDENT:

Miss Midway, an intermediate-level student, reported to the head nurse that a two-year-old child she was caring for had a temperature elevation of 103.4° F. It was noted that the nurse had not lifted the side rails on the crib after she had taken the child's temperature.

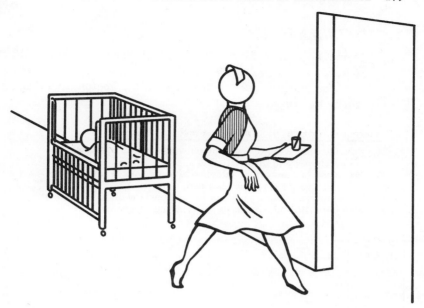

4. Meeting the patient's physical and medical needs
   a. Made error in giving medication, treatment, or other nursing care.
   b. Ignored or failed to carry out orders.
   c. Overlooked need for improvement or safety in environment.
   d. Caused patient discomfort due to lack of skill, awkwardness.
   e. Did not prepare patient properly for test, treatment, procedure.

2/16	4c	*Left side rail down on crib*

This is an incident of ineffective behavior. Even though the student noti-fied the head nurse about the fact that there was an elevation in the child's temperature (and this was important and the right thing to do), she over-looked the environmental safety of her patient. A young child with a tem-perature elevation might be irrational and could fall out of a crib. Moreover, the side rails should always be elevated on every crib before the nurse leaves the bedside under any circumstances. The appropriate classification for this incident would be 4c, "Overlooked need for improvement or *safety* in environment."

INCIDENT:

Miss Older, an advanced-level student, placed a newly admitted patient who was having respiratory distress in an orthopneic position and remained with him until the doctor and inhalation therapist arrived.

4. Meeting the patient's physical and medical needs

    A. Carried out medical order or nursing care procedure correctly despite difficulties.
    B. Made use of comfort or nursing care measures until medical orders could be obtained.
    C. Make environmental changes for patient's welfare or safety.
    D. Was very skillful or gentle in giving nursing care.

2/2	4B	Put pt. in orthopneic pos.

Often upon admission of a patient, the nurse will find the patient has certain problems that require immediate nursing care. In this instance Miss Older's experience indicated recall of the appropriate action to take when a patient has respiratory distress (with no indication of special attention or care to be given). In this instance the patient had just been admitted, therefore it was too early for doctors' orders to be available. Miss Older acted quickly to apply her knowledge and placed the patient in an orthopneic position to ease his breathing until the doctor and therapist arrived. This is an effective behavior and should be classified under 4 B, "Made use of comfort or nursing care measures until medical orders could be obtained."

Behavior Area 5
Applying Scientific Principles to Nursing Care

In this area the nurse must demonstrate capability in the application of scientific principles in practical situations. Specific circumstances may require special handling. Thus rote memorization of the principle will not be enough; the nurse must be able to apply the principle to solve the immediate problem.

INCIDENT:

Miss Midway, an intermediate-level student, was caring for a patient who had developed a staphylococcic infection of his

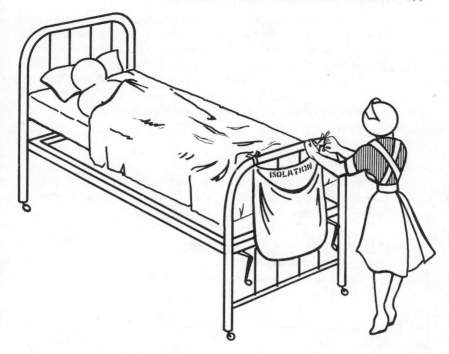

incision. It was observed that she placed his bed linens in an isolation bag, even though no order had been written for isolation.

5. Applying scientific principles to nursing care
   A. Exhibited understanding of advanced nursing principles.
   B. Questioned situation which violated underlying principles.

3/6	5B	Used isolation bag / Staph. case

This was an effective incident in which the student recalled and applied information about the scientific principles involved in avoiding the spread of infection. She used her initiative and judgment, even though she was not specifically directed to do so, and she placed the soiled linens in an isolation bag. The action prevented the spread of infection. This incident should be classified under 5B, "Questioned situation which violated underlying principles." In this instance the nurse did more than question the matter in her mind; she did something about it, based on her knowledge of what to do.

If the same situation had confronted a first-level student who was alert to the fact that this was a situation involving infection, it is possible that she would sense the need for some kind of protective measure, but may not yet have learned how to handle the problem. In the case of a first-level student if she had not already learned about the use of isolation bags for the linens of patients with infections, the appropriate action might have been for her to ask the head nurse what to do with the linens before she began changing the patient's bed.

INCIDENT:

Miss Young, a first-level student, was observed wearing a black woolen sweater while giving a bed bath to a patient with an upper respiratory infection.

5. Applying scientific principles to nursing care
   a. Did not know vital theory or principles of nursing care.
   b. Ignored or failed to apply scientific principles.

2/4	5b	Wore sweater on Ward

In this situation there would be two factors: (1) It is not appropriate for a nurse to wear a sweater with her uniform when giving patient care. This is a matter of professional grooming. However, a more serious point is involved: (2) Wool tends to attract and hold microorganisms. This tends to cause the spread of infection from one patient to another and is a violation of basic scientific principles. In this instance the more serious matter is the danger to other patients through the violation of scientific principles. The classification would be 5b, "Ignored or failed to apply scientific principles."

Behavior Area 6
Observing, Reporting, and Charting

Observing and reporting are two independent skills, but it would be difficult to assess them as separate behaviors. A nurse may be alert to patient needs, but if she has poor communication skills, she may not remember to report what she has observed. The instructor should investigate the behavior of students in this area to ascertain where they may be having difficulty; whether it involves better knowledge and checking on patient needs, or whether it is a matter of recording and reporting facts the nurse has observed.

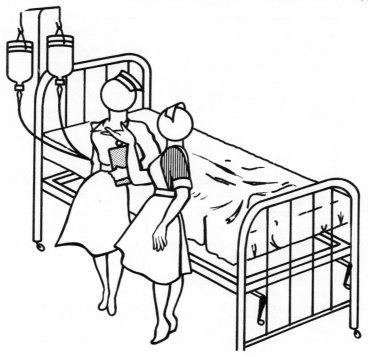

INCIDENT:

Miss Young, a first-level student, during a routine check, noted that a patient who was receiving a blood transfusion was having a chill. She stopped the flow of blood, but did not remove the needle from the vein. She immediately notified the instructor and the doctor.

6. Observing, reporting, and charting

    A. Noticed and reported special physical, emotional, or social need of patient.
    B. Immediately reported new symptoms or significant change.
    C. Reported why medication or treatment could not be given.
    D. Reported significant facts to relief nurse.
    E. Wrote excellent nurse's notes.

3/18	6B	Stopped transf. / reported chill

This is an effective incident. In this case the student checked on the patient's condition and observed a significant sign, a chill. She immediately stopped the flow of blood. This was effective. She then immediately reported to the instructor and the doctor. She did not remove the needle since under ordinary circumstances she is not authorized to do so without an order. This was also effective. The appropriate classification for the incident would be 6 B, "Immediately reported new symptoms or significant change."

INCIDENT:

Miss Older, an advanced-level student, recorded the vital signs on the chart of a patient whose diagnosis was subarachnoid hemorrhage. In charting, she recognized there was a marked deviation in the pulse from that taken 15 minutes previously. She proceeded with other patient care assignments.

6. Observing, reporting, and charting
   a. Failed to notice need for special patient care.
   b. Failed to report significant facts about patient's condition.
   c. Failed to report off duty or to report unfinished patient care.
   d. Failed to chart treatment, observations, or nursing care.
   e. Charted or transcribed incorrectly or incompletely.

1/10	6 b	*No report on pulse change*

This is an ineffective incident. Here was a case where the nurse noted a deviation in a pulse rate for a patient for whom this was particularly significant. She should have notified the head nurse or a doctor at once about the change in pulse rate. This would be classified as 6b, "Failure to report significant facts about patient's condition." Merely charting the change was not sufficient.

Behavior Area 7
Adaptability to New or Stressful Situations

Behavior in emergency situations or capability in handling contingencies is important. Many situations cause stress: close supervision, heavy patient load, tension between nurse and patient, or poor interpersonal relations between members of the staff. Sometimes the pressures are self-imposed, as in instances where students are concerned about personal problems and find it difficult to concentrate on assignments on the ward. Another aspect of this behavior area is the nurse's ability to cope with the unexpected or new situation. Regardless of the amount of education a nurse may acquire, there will still be some things she may not have encountered before in a learning situation, but which she must face in performing nursing care. For this reason, the nurse should be sufficiently flexible that she has the ability to cope with emergency situations, or to handle the new or un-expected turn of events. Problem-solving is an important skill in this area.

INCIDENT:

Miss Midway, an intermediate-level student, answered a signal light and found she had been summoned by an ambulatory pa-tient sharing the room with a patient who was convulsing. The nurse immediately placed a tongue blade in the mouth of the convulsing patient, lifted the side rails on his bed, and sum-moned the intern. She also assured the ambulatory patient that the convulsion would subside in a few minutes.

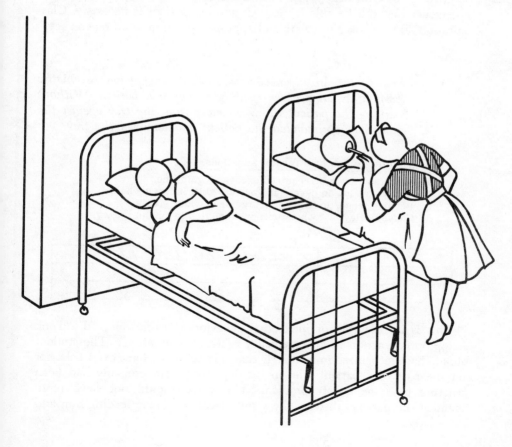

7. Adaptability to new or stressful situations

    A. Required minimum guidance in adjusting to new situation.
    B. Learned new procedure or skill quickly.
    C. Carried out nursing care calmly and efficiently under stress.
    D. Took immediate and appropriate action in an emergency.

3/21	7 D	Gave aid in convulsion / Called Dr.

This is an effective incident. A number of factors are involved here. First is the nurse's ability to take appropriate action immediately: She placed a tongue blade in the patient's mouth, thereby maintaining a patent airway. She recognized the limitations of her ability to relieve the patient's symptoms and summoned the assistance of an intern. She also had a responsibility to the ambulatory patient who reacted when he observed the severity of the convulsion. The nurse should be able to act quickly in an emergency and still be able to reassure another patient if necessary. Classification, 7D, "Took immediate and appropriate action in an emergency."

INCIDENT:

Miss Older, an advanced-level student, during her psychiatric learning experience was feeding a depressed patient. Without warning the patient threw a saucer from the tray against the wall. She reprimanded the patient and removed the tray.

7. Adaptability to new or stressful situations

    a. Adjusted slowly or required excessive guidance.
    b. Was very slow in developing manual skill in new technique.
    c. Became tense, upset, or disorganized under stress.
    d. Caused delay or took inappropriate action in an emergency.

1/25	7c	Scolded depressed pt.

This is an example of ineffective behavior. Classification, 7d, "Took inappropriate action in an emergency" (stressful situation). The student should have recognized immediately that this was an extreme overt behavior on the part of a patient who in his depressed state probably had been reacting to some covert problem. The nurse should not have reprimanded the patient. Instead, she should have continued feeding him and should have continued endeavoring to establish and maintain rapport with him. She should not have shown evidence of being disturbed by removing the patient's tray.

Behavior Area 8
Relations with Co-Workers, Physicians, and Visitors

Many a technically competent person finds it difficult to relate to other people—co-workers, superiors, and others. In the nursing situation it is important to keep lines of communication open and free and to be able to interact favorably with people at all levels. Personal moods, dislikes, or other problems should not interfere with the performance of nursing care and interaction with others in the nursing situation. Personnel in the hospital must work together with a minimum of friction. Every nurse has a responsibility to make certain that she does nothing to contribute to tensions or unfavorable interpersonal relationships, whether they involve other members of the staff, the patient, or visitors.

INCIDENT:

Miss Older, an advanced-level student, was observed giving instruction about the positioning of a footboard to a new practical nurse.

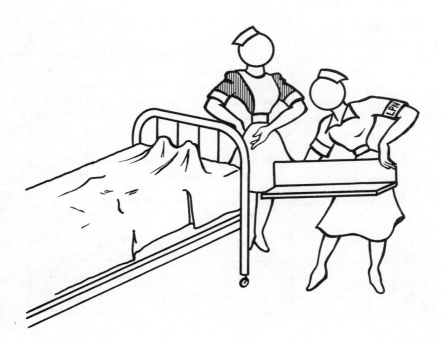

8. Relations with co-workers, physicians, and visitors

    A. Was tactful in handling difficult situation.

    B. Was cooperative with co-workers, physicians, other personnel.

    C. Assisted in instruction and supervision of auxiliary personnel.

2/17	8C	*Taught L.P.N. to apply ft. bd.*

Auxiliary personnel often must perform procedures for which guidance and supervision are needed. A nurse must be willing and alert to opportunities to assist others in a subordinate role to give patient care. In this case, a new practical nurse was attempting to insert a footboard for patient comfort. If the student noted any difficulty, she should have taken occasion to assist and instruct the L.P.N. Good interpersonal skills are needed in this situation because the student nurse may be a very young person, whereas the practical nurse may be somewhat older, or the student may be short and the L.P.N. tall (or there could be other differences the student would have to handle with tact and diplomacy, showing ability to maintain good interpersonal relationships).

INCIDENT:

Miss Midway, an intermediate-level student, was caring for a chronically ill patient whose daughter had cared for him in their home for seven years. The daughter suggested a deviation in the routine procedure being performed by the nurse. She said it would make the patient more comfortable. The student informed the daughter that she had been properly educated as a nurse to care for this type of patient and asked the daughter to step out of the room.

8. Relations with co-workers, physicians, and visitors

    a. Was tactless or rude to visitor or hospital personnel.

    b. Failed to cooperate with co-workers or others.

    c. Did not use opportunity for teaching auxiliary personnel.

    d. Interfered with instruction, supervision, or work of others.

2/7	8a	*Was rude to pt's daughter*

This is an example of an ineffective behavior. It would be classified under 8a, "Was tactless or rude to visitor." In order to establish good interpersonal relationships the student should have recognized that the daughter had cared for the patient for a number of years and would know about measures that had provided for his comfort. It is true the student has been taught to perform procedures correctly; however, she has at the same time been taught to be flexible, resourceful, and realistic if need be when certain situations arise. Her attitude and the manner in which she dismissed the patient's daughter from the room were contraindicated. By this behavior the student no doubt lost rapport with the daughter, who was visiting, and probably with the patient as well due to her abrupt manner. Rudeness and lack of tact are not acceptable in nursing.

Behavior Area 9
Judgment Regarding Professional Values

This area involves behaviors in the affective domain, those of personal and professional values. Honesty, forthrightness, acceptance of personal responsibility for errors, awareness of ethical codes, and respect for the confidence of others are some of the specific values involved here.

INCIDENT:

Miss Midway, an intermediate-level student, noted that the order on the medication card differed from the order on the Kardex and doctor's orders. This was not a new order. However, the student refused to give the medication until the situation was clarified.

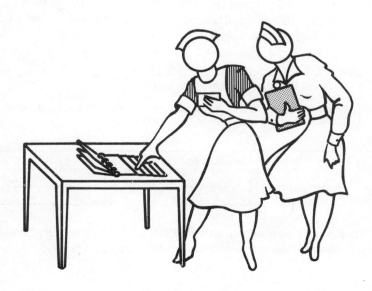

9. Judgment regarding professional values
    A. Called attention to own error which was otherwise unnoticed.
    B. Reported situation accurately despite reflection on self.
    C. Kept information confidential despite pressure to divulge it.
    D. Maintained ethical standards in a difficult situation.

2/7	9D	*Req. Clarif. of med. Order*

This is an example of maintaining a standard of professional values in a difficult situation. The order was not new; this could imply that others had followed it. The student could have assumed since no one else had questioned or noted the discrepancy that she could follow suit. However, the student did note the discrepancy and before giving medication (which may have been the improper dosage), she insisted on a clarification of the matter. This was an effective behavior in area 9D, "Maintained ethical standards in a difficult situation."

At first glance it may appear that the item could be classified under 2D, "Noting inconsistency in medication." It is true an inconsistency was noted, but in this instance more was involved—an ethical issue. The student maintained her stand against giving a dose which could have been incorrect and harmful to the patient. She asked for specific orders with clarification of a conflict.

INCIDENT:

Miss Young, a first-level student, informed the patient that his diagnostic test results thus far were all normal except the x-ray findings of the stomach.

9. Judgment regarding professional values
    a. Tried to cover up or denied obvious error.
    b. Made exaggerated statements about nursing care given.
    c. Used poor judgment about releasing confidential information.
    d. Used questionable judgment in ethical matter.

3/7	9c	*Released Conf. info to pt.*

This would be classified as an ineffective incident—area 9c, "Used poor judgment about releasing confidential information." The nurse is not authorized to give medical information unless she is instructed to do so. This is the doctor's responsibility. The nurse may prepare the patient for a treatment he is to receive by informing him that the treatment will take place, provided such treatment has been ordered and will take place. The nurse may brief the patient to prepare him psychologically for the treatment. However, she is not authorized to give medical information or information about the diagnosis. In this case the nurse merely created a situation in which there could be increased anxiety. A nurse must be aware constantly of the need for exercising good judgment about the manner in which she answers the patients' questions. Answers to patients should be comforting but should indicate that an effort will be made to have the doctor answer such questions as soon as possible. The nurse should indicate neither positive nor negative information before the physician has had an opportunity to talk with the patient.

Behavior Area 10
Use of Learning Opportunities

In a ward experience, which is truly educational, the student can take advantage of many learning opportunities. She has an opportunity to learn about patients' diagnoses, to study the medical care plan and its effect on the patients' prognoses. There are opportunities to observe new techniques, to participate in conferences with doctors, social workers, dietitians, and other members of the health team. This can provide good learning experiences with chances to seek clarification and instruction.

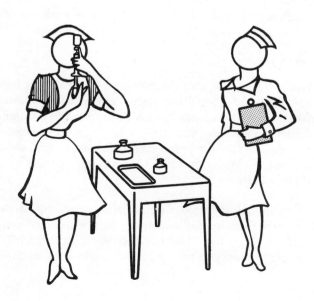

INCIDENT:

Miss Young, a first-level student, noted a first-day postopera-
tive appendectomy patient was having considerable pain. She
checked the Kardex and noted there was a p.r.n. narcotic order
for pain. She also noted he had received a narcotic six hours
earlier. She reported this to the instructor and asked for super-
vision on the administration of the narcotic.

10. Use of learning opportunities
    A. Made significant contribution to ward conference.
    B. Expended extra effort to follow through on patient care.
    C. Asked to observe or learn a new procedure.
    D. Accepted suggestions and criticism graciously.
    E. Asked for supervision or guidance when needed.

2/20	10 E	*Asked help c̄ Narcotic*

This is an effective behavior. Possibly the first inclination would be to
classify this as an incident of checking. It is true the nurse did check on the
Kardex for orders in response to the patient's condition. However, there
is another important point. This was a first-level student, and it was the
first time she was attempting to administer a narcotic. The fact that she
asked for supervision was an effective behavior. The appropriate classification for this behavior would be 10E, "Asked for supervision or guidance
when needed."

INCIDENT:

Miss Midway, an intermediate-level student, was assigned the
leader role for a ward conference one week in advance. When
the conference took place, Miss Midway could not guide the dis-
cussion because she was unprepared. When the instructor asked
her why she was not prepared for the conference, she stated she
had not had time to study the material because of all of her
other activities.

This is a case of lack of preparation on the part of the student which
prevented her from participating effectively in a ward conference. There
are two possibilities—(1) 10a, "Did not participate in or prepare for ward
conference" is the appropriate area; (2) 10d might have been considered

10. Use of learning opportunities
   a. Did not participate in or prepare for ward conference.
   b. Failed to keep clinical records up to date.
   c. Failed to take advantage of opportunity to learn.
   d. Was defensive, indignant, or indifferent about criticism.
   e. Failed to ask for guidance or went to improper authority.

2/4	10 a	*Unprepared for ward conf.*

depending on the degree of defensiveness the student displayed in placing the blame on the fact that she was overloaded with other activities.

Students should learn to regard ward conferences as learning opportunities and should prepare for participation anytime one is scheduled. Often the student puts too much emphasis on the preparation of other assignments and neglects preparation for ward conference because she does not give this kind of assignment sufficient priority or importance in her study plan. All opportunities for learning experiences are important, and the nursing student should make adequate preparation for each one in turn.

Behavior Area 11
Acceptance of Nursing Service Responsibility

In this area there may be differences from one school to another in relation to the degree of responsibility the nursing student can assume. Once the nurse becomes a registered practitioner, there is no problem; she is then responsible for the full share of nursing care. However, a student should regard each assignment on the ward as an opportunity to grow and develop in her capability for assuming responsibilities for patient care. Some desirable habits of responsibility the student can cultivate include promptness, a sense of economy and regard for hospital equipment and property, a willingness to accept and follow organizational policy, a willingness to accept extra assignments or changes of schedule necessitated by emergency situations. The skills important in this area include leadership and management.

INCIDENT:

Miss Older, an advanced-level student, was functioning as a team leader on Ward C. She was observed delegating different tasks to the various levels of team members during the team conference and explaining the general problem to the group so

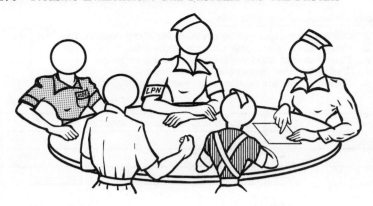

that each member of the team understood his share of responsibility.

11. Acceptance of nursing service responsibility

    A. Voluntarily assumed extra duties within limits of responsibility.
    B. Willingly cooperated with assignment or schedule change.
    C. Followed established policy or procedure despite difficulties.
    D. Assumed leadership or management responsibilities as needed.
    E. Took care to conserve supplies and equipment.

3/1	11D	*Deleg. team tasks & expl.*

This is an incident of effective behavior in acceptance of responsibility. The appropriate classification would be 11D, "Assumed leadership or management responsibility as needed." As a third-level student, she had reached the point in her educational program where she should be able to delegate assignments to members of the nursing team. Nurses must be able to assume this kind of responsibility which involves not only the delegation of responsibility to others, but the ability to define clearly what each member of the team must do, to follow through to see that each one carries out the assignment, and to make changes or modifications in the plan as needed.

INCIDENT:

Miss Older, an advanced-level student, sent a nurse's aide to the pharmacy with a narcotic vial for a stock refill.

This is an incident of ineffective behavior in assuming nursing service responsibility—area 11c. Miss Older deviated from the established policy.

11. Acceptance of nursing service responsibility
   a. Ignored or refused task beyond assignment or responsibilities.
   b. Was uncooperative in schedule or assignment change.
   c. Deviated from established policy or procedure.
   d. Arrived on department unnecessarily late.
   e. Wasted, destroyed, or damaged supplies or equipment.

12/19	11 c	Sent aide to get narcotic

In the first analysis the refilling of stock narcotics is the responsibility of the registered professional nurse. In the second place, delegating this responsibility to a nurse's aide is a gross error since narcotics may be handled only by authorized personnel, and a nurse's aide is not among the personnel authorized to handle narcotics.

Behavior Area 12
Personal Appearance

A minimum standard of good grooming is expected of every nurse. This is a standard commensurate with professional requirements and uniform conduct. In this situation behaviors that are not routine but rather unusual, depending on the circumstances, would be regarded as ineffective.

INCIDENT:

Miss Midway, an intermediate-level student, had been spattered with blood while helping the doctor with an emergency case. She asked for permission to go to change her apron before giving care to the next patient.

12. Personal appearance

   A. Made change in grooming which improved personal appearance.

2/12	12 A	asked perm. to ch. apron

This is an example of effective behavior and consideration of personal appearance for the esthetic effect on patients and others who see the nurse. It should be classified as 12A, "Made changes in grooming which improved personal appearance."

INCIDENT:

An instructor observed the poor posture of Miss Midway, an intermediate-level student, 5'11" tall. The instructor discussed the problem with her. Miss Midway was later observed making a special effort to stand and walk erectly following the counseling session.

Here is an example of a student complying with a constructive suggestion regarding personal appearance. Often it is difficult to make changes in personal habits. The nursing student must be willing to do this, particularly if the adoption of a new habit will improve personal appearance. In addition, the student should be aware of and practice the principles of good body mechanics, especially in the hospital setting.

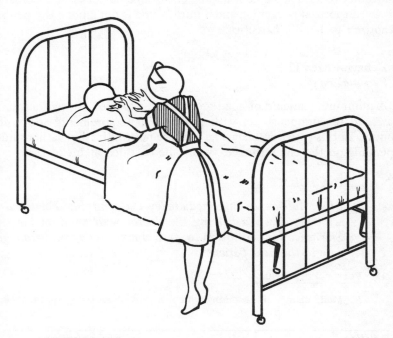

INCIDENT:

Miss Midway, an intermediate-level student, was observed giving back care to a convalescent patient. The patient complained of an irritation and a scratching sensation. The instructor observed the nurse was wearing an engagement ring, also that the student's nails were very long and sharp.

12. Personal appearance
    a. Failed to wear uniform as required.
    b. Appeared untidy, not well groomed.

1/15	12a	Wore ring ō setting

This is an example of an ineffective incident in personal grooming. A nurse should make certain her nails are well groomed, but not sharp and pointed to the extent that they might cause scratching or irritation to a patient's skin. It is not desirable to wear rings with stone settings when giving patient care. Sharp edges on rings can cause irritation when the nurse is rubbing the skin surface of a patient's back, for example. In addition, rings, jewelry, or adornments other than a wedding band are considered a violation of uniform regulations.

USING EVALUATION
TO PLAN FOR PROGRESS

How can the record be used for student guidance? Is the record a rating device? How long should the record be kept?

Planning for Progress

The most important benefit deriving from the use of the Clinical Experience Record is the information it provides for student guidance. The record presents a graphic picture of the trends of behavior to be encouraged and those to be improved. The incidents on the record should be studied by the instructor to determine whether there is a significant pattern in a particular area. If the instructor notes several instances of ineffective behavior in the same area or in related areas, this should be used as the basis for planning for remedial action.

Progress reviews should be scheduled periodically with each student. The progress review is a private interview between the instructor and the student at which time the student's performance record is discussed in detail.

The most distinguishing feature about the use of the critical incident procedures for evaluation is the fact that the record belongs not to the observer or instructor alone, it belongs jointly to the instructor and the student. Together they share in "writing" the record. The student performs assignments to the best of her ability; the instructor observes critical incidents that occur. They share the responsibility for using the record constructively. Thus, at intervals throughout a clinical experience the instructor and the student should meet to discuss the record and its implications. On the basis of the critical incidents on the record they should plan for progress or they should arrange for remedial action.

Consider the following suggestions in planning for progress:

1. Define the Student's Personal Goals
Get to know each student. Each one is different; each may have a different goal in attending the school. You as an instructor should help each student to establish realistic goals consistent with the student's capabilities.

2. Identify the Student as an Individual
No student likes to be just one of a group without an individual identity. As early as possible in the clinical serve or semester try to learn each student's name and use the name when you address that student. Try to create the feeling that it is important to be John Regan or Mary McLain who hopes one day to become a professional nurse. Each is important as a student and as a potential nurse. Each eventually will represent your school of nursing.

3. Help the Student to Identify Problems
A good knowledge of the student will enable you to help to identify problems. It is not suggested that you solve the student's problems— you should help the student to solve his or her own problems.

Lead the student to a discussion of the problems. Concentrate on problems in relation to status as a student. Do not attempt to probe into personal problems unless it becomes apparent that they are interfering with the student's progress. Try to get the student to offer solutions to the problems. If the solutions she offers are clearly unreasonable or inconsistent, offer suggestions for alternate actions.

4. Schedule Progress Reviews Periodically
These reviews should be held—
a. When the student's performance indicates there is need for a review;
b. When the student feels help is needed;
c. Periodically throughout the clinical serve or semester.

How to Conduct a Progress Review
Try to follow a careful pattern in conducting the progress review. Remember the purpose of the review is to plan for improvement and progress.

1. *Keep the objectives of the interview in mind.*
2. *Schedule the interview in advance* and inform the student of the time.

3. *Hold the interview in privacy,* away from other students and other people who may know the student.
4. *Try to avoid interruptions.*
5. *Establish contact with the student.* Place the student at ease. Endeavor, if possible, to let the student introduce some of the points of discussion. This helps to establish rapport. Some students will resist the interview and may tend to be uneasy and rigid in the interview situation. Try to eliminate this problem.
6. *Open the discussion on a positive note* and *maintain a positive approach.* Try to commend the student for the effective behaviors on her record first. This will help to create a pleasant atmosphere. Try to maintain a positive approach throughout the interview, even though there may be a necessity for bringing up the discussion of ineffective behaviors.
7. *Avoid blaming the student* for ineffective behaviors. This may come as a surprise. It is not desirable to fix blame. It is far better to attempt to *identify the reasons for the behavior* rather than to blame the student because it occurred. In this way it is possible to help the student to recognize the problem and to plan to overcome it.
8. *Encourage the student to discuss why the problem exists.* Often you will find the student does not realize there is a problem, or perhaps views the problem in the wrong light. Encourage a discussion of why ineffective incidents occurred from the student's point of view.
9. *Emphasize the confidential nature of the interview.* Keep in mind that the information discussed in the interview is private. Assure the student that the information will not be discussed with others.
10. *Avoid reference to other students.* Comparisons accomplish very little. No student likes to be compared with a rival. Avoid gossip or hearsay about the behavior of others. The important topic is the student with whom you are holding the interview.
11. *Discuss personal problems only if they relate to the situation.* Try to avoid becoming the student's confidante for personal problems. Often a student will suffer the anguish of having discussed a personal problem which she would prefer to keep to herself. Be extremely careful in encouraging discussions of personal problems. An instructor can learn to handle this situation diplomatically without turning the student away in times of need. It should be fairly easy to identify situations in which the student is seeking assistance as distinguished from situations in which students tend to make you a surrogate "mother." Often the experience of being away from home for the first time will in itself create a personal problem for the student. She may be homesick, she may feel inadequate, or she may not be able to relate to the other students readily. The alert instructor should be able to sense these problems and encourage the

student to discuss them. Conversely, there will be students who grow too dependent and who will want to unburden all their problems on your shoulders.

When a student enrolls in a school of nursing, one of the experiences she must face is growing up, and in doing so she must learn to cope with her own problems. You will do a student a great service if you encourage her to accept and assume responsibility for her own problems.

12. *Help to build satisfaction and pride in the student.* Nursing is a proud profession, and any student who enrolls in a school of nursing should develop a sense of pride and satisfaction in the career ahead. A sense of self-realization and self-satisfaction in one's choice of a career can become a motivating factor in achieving objectives. Whenever possible, take occasion to build this sense of satisfaction.

13. *Be patient.* Changes will not occur overnight. An instructor must have a great deal of patience and be willing to wait for changes in behavior to occur. Poor personal habits are difficult to overcome, but with the right kind of guidance a student can be assisted in overcoming them. Inability to communicate can be an item of ineffective behavior on the student's record. It takes time to overcome this kind of problem. Encourage any positive signs of improvement that you note. Help the student to recognize signs of improvement in her own behavior. If there is no evidence of progress after the initial interview, review the problem again and try to establish a better basis for improvement. Sometimes the student misses the point the first time. Be patient—try to help as much as necessary.

14. *Identify lack of motivation and poor attitudes.* At times you will find students who do not respond. They show no sign of improvement following a progress review, nor do they indicate any interest in improving their behavior. This type of student may have several problems. There may be a lack of motivation because of a lack of interest in becoming a nurse. If this is the case, a real problem exists. Identify the basic problem first. If the student is enrolled in the school of nursing just to please her parents, or someone else, she may never reach the goal. The nature of nursing requires dedication and a very high degree of motivation. Therefore people who have no interest in nursing should not be encouraged to continue. Students like this should be identified as early as possible and should be encouraged to seek other fields of education.

On the other hand, you may encounter a student who does want to become a nurse who may have attitudes that are not appropriate for nursing. Changing basic attitudes about people and about hard work, long hours, and heavy assignments may take time. If a student expects to become an effective nurse, she must develop the appropriate set of attitudes about nursing.

15. Close the interview on a *note of continuity and interest.* Even though the student has many ineffective behaviors on her record, attempt to close the interview on a hopeful and constructive note. Suggest that the student give some thought to the plans you and she have made and that she try to improve in the areas where there are problems. Encourage her to look forward to the next interview when she will be able to see the progress she has made. Close the discussion with a comment such as "We seem to have a good set of plans, let's see how much you can accomplish during the next few weeks. Feel free to come to me when you need to discuss the problems we have talked about."

If the progress review is conducted along the lines suggested above, it should serve as a very constructive portion of the student's educational program. The Clinical Experience Record serves not only as the basis for initiating improvement, but as the basis for showing when improvement takes place. As the student's behavior improves, there should be critical incidents of an effective nature recorded on the form. If she continues to improve, the trend should become apparent by the notations of a number of effective incidents in an area where ineffective behaviors had been recorded in an earlier period. Show the student the transition, and commend her for the improvement.

The Clinical Experience Record form can be used (1) to identify strengths and weaknesses, (2) to indicate growing trends of behavior that should be encouraged or corrected, (3) as a basis for guidance and counseling, (4) as a reference form for new instructors, (5) as a source of information for developing an over-all evaluation for purposes of references for employment following graduation.

Is the Clinical Experience Record a Rating Device?

The purpose of the performance record procedures is to summarize critical incidents of behavior on the basis of observations made by instructors and others who are in a position to observe the performance of students and practitioners. It is not possible to subtract ineffective incidents from effective incidents and arrive at a grade or rating. No percentage points can be assigned to the various areas of behavior, nor should there be any attempt to summarize the record in the form of an over-all grade by designations such as Outstanding, Good, Fair, Poor.

The Clinical Experience Record is intended to supplement other kinds of evaluative information such as test scores, class presentations, outside assignments, and special projects. No single factor should constitute the basis for a grade—all aspects of the student's performance should be taken into consideration. If the student does an outstanding job in class work and written assignments but is unable to perform well in clinical areas as evidenced by ineffective behaviors recorded on her Clinical Experience

Record, this information should be taken into consideration in assigning a value grade to the student's performance.

The most efficient way to advise the student of her performance is to provide information that will be much more meaningful than a mere letter such as A, B, or C. A student is able to learn very little from this type of grade. On the other hand, if she is informed that her class work and written assignments were excellent, however, her performance in clinical areas was ineffective in the manner in which she communicated with patients, and in her failure to apply scientific principles to practical situations, the student has a basis for working to improve her behavior. She has definite indication of the areas of weakness. At the same time, she realizes that the instructor recognized and gave her credit for the class work and outside assignments which were of high quality.

When used to supplement other information about student activities and performance, the Clinical Experience Record can be a very effective evaluation tool. It serves not only as a record of facts about performance but as a basis for both the instructor and student to plan toward improvement and progress.

Other Uses of the Clinical Experience Record

One of the many purposes served by the performance record is its value as a cumulative record. The Clinical Experience Record forms should be placed in a cumulative file after each clinical serve. In this way it will be possible for anyone reviewing records to gain insight into the nature of performance over the period of several clinical serves and several semesters. A glance back at several Clinical Experience Records in the student's file can help to identify over-all trends which may be significant from the standpoint of special areas of interest the student may develop. It is possible to note gradual development and growth from the cumulative information provided in a series of Clinical Experience Records.

Much important information can be gathered from a survey of the Clinical Experience Records of a group of students. Instructors will note clusters of behaviors in certain areas at times. This may indicate the need for a review of the methods used to teach certain aspects of the course. If there are numerous occurrences of ineffective behavior in the application of scientific principles for most of the students in the group, it should begin to be evident to the instructor that most of the students failed to grasp the need to adapt what they learned in the classroom or in the laboratory to the practical situation on the ward. This should be one way to collect information that can lead to improvement in the teaching program. Feedback of this type not only is important to the students in pointing out problems in learning, it is also valuable in pinpointing problems in instruction.

One of the important uses of the Clinical Experience Record from an administrative and instructional point of view is for summarizing student performance for employment purposes. When over-all evaluations of capability are requested by future employers, this information can be summarized efficiently and quickly from the student's Clinical Experience Record, with specific indications of strengths and weaknesses.

Bibliography

Flanagan, John C., Gosnell, Doris, and Fivars, Grace. "Evaluating Student Performance," *Am. J. Nursing,* 63: 96-99, (Nov.) 1963.

Flanagan, John C., Marchese, Angeline C., Tuska, Shirley A., and Fivars, Grace. *Instructor's Manual for the Clinical Experience Record for Nursing Students,* Psychometric Techniques Associates, Pittsburgh, 1960.

Selected References

Coker, Robert, Gosnell, Doris, and Hart, Frances. "Public Health in the Nursing School," *Public Health Reports,* 72:325-28, (April) 1957.

Dunlap, Marjorie. "The Development of Professional Graduate Program of Nursing," unpublished doctoral dissertation, University of Southern California, 1959.

Glaser, Robert, and Klaus, David. "Proficiency Measurement: Assessing Human Performance," chapter in *Psychological Principles in System Development,* Robert M. Gagné (ed.), Holt, Rinehart, and Winston, Inc., New York, 1962.

Hoffman, Katherine J. "A Suggested Method for the Development of a Tool to Aid in the Evaluation of Performance in Nursing," unpublished doctoral dissertation, University of Washington, 1956.

Nurse Utilization Project Staff. *An Investigation of the Relation between Nursing Activity and Patient Welfare,* Iowa State University, 1960.

Rosenberg, P. P., and Fuller, M. "Dynamic Analysis of the Student Nurse," *Group Psychotherapy,* 10:22-37, 1957.

Critical Incident

The Director of Nursing Service met with a committee of the Nursing Service Organization—the Committee on Personnel Practice. She had asked each member of the group previous to the meeting to review her job description in relation to the functions and qualifications as designated in the ANA Statement of their respective positions. During the course of the meeting the group reviewed the organizational plan of the nursing service department. It was noted by a supervisor in the group that the licensed practical nurse was omitted from the plan.

Two effective incidents stand out: (1) The supervisor noticed an omission on the organizational plan of the licensed practical nurse. (2) The Director of Nursing Service was involving appropriate personnel in an evaluation of job descriptions in relation to accepted standards.

Standard #4 of "Standards for Organized Nursing Services" (ANA) states: "The nursing department's organizational plan delineates the functional structure of the nursing department and shows relationships of personnel."

The Director of Nursing Service, in group session, was stimulating the Committee on Personnel Practice to assess the factors necessary to conform to an accepted standard of practice. This type of behavior, if properly channeled, will no doubt lead to assessment of another factor under Standard #8 (e) "a written job description is available to each member of the nursing department."

Chapter 10

Evaluation in

Terms of

Professional Standards

In a brief span of years nursing has moved to take its place among the health professions. The Florence Nightingale Pledge remains our credo, reinforced now by the Code of Ethics for the Nursing Profession. Standards for Organized Nursing Services* have been established by the American Nurses Association to provide professional guidelines for nursing in health facilities in any environment: hospitals, public health agencies, nursing homes, industrial settings, and other health clinics.

A mark of distinction in any profession is its ability to police itself with respect to standards. The establishment of standards for nursing is a "first step toward . . . efficiency"† in offering the kinds of service needed to meet the demands of society and the changing world and at the same time satisfy the needs of the professional practitioner. The standards are flexible and can be revised and modified to adapt to the constantly changing economic, social, and political scene. It is the intent of leaders at the national level who established the standards to initiate their use as a means for measuring performance. It is the further intent of the national committees that these standards be upheld and maintained as the bench marks for the nursing profession. It remains with each nurse to practice in a manner consistent with the established standards, and for each head nurse and others in supervisory capacities to insist on performance to meet this quality.

We now have the basis on which to establish objectives for performance not only at the student level, but successively from the school to the bedside and beyond to the health facilities of the community in the

* "Standards for Organized Nursing Services," *Am. J. Nursing*, 65:76-79, (March) 1965.
† *Am. J. Nursing, loc. cit.*

industrial and clinical environment. The National League for Nursing has developed criteria for the achievement of the established standards.* The rest is up to us!

IT IS OUR MOVE

Standardizing agencies, educators, and others have led the way; the responsibility now becomes a matter of local concern. Each hospital and health agency must redefine its standards in terms of its facility. Each faculty committee in schools of nursing must redefine educational objectives in terms of national standards.

Standards of acceptable performance can now be established consistent with the criteria developed by the League. The Standards for Organized Nursing Services provide the basis for the development of professional policy relating to administrative control, personnel practices, over-all hospital or health facility organization, and most important, nursing care to the patient.

What Can the Critical Incident Contribute to Meeting Standards?

Can the Clinical Experience Record program help to implement the standards set forth by the American Nurses Association and the criteria developed by the National League for Nursing? The way is clear for the initiation and conduct of a program for evaluation in terms of the accomplishment of stated objectives. Once these have been defined in behavioral terms describing acceptable nursing performance, the program can proceed. The critical incident technique can be used to collect facts and as a basis for evaluating the effectiveness of performance. Where standards are part of the general body of knowledge and information, and where practitioners responsible for nursing care and those responsible for management and the operation of a health facility are in accord, the Clinical Experience Record program can be used to evaluate performance in terms of professional standards. Effectiveness can now be measured at all levels in terms of recognized standards—criteria for better nursing care.

We've come a long way from Scutari!

Bibliography

American Nurses Association. "Standards for Organized Nursing Services," *Am. J. Nursing,* 65:76-79, (March) 1965.
National League for Nursing. *Criteria for Evaluating a Hospital Department of Nursing Service,* Department of Hospital Nursing, National League for Nursing, New York, 1965.

* *Criteria for Evaluating a Hospital Department of Nursing Service,* Dept. of Hospital Nursing, National League for Nursing, New York, 1965.

Appendix I
Critical Requirements
for Selected Fields

**Critical Requirements
for Case Workers
(Social Work)***

   I. Assessing client problem and the relevance of agency services to
meet it
     A. Securing an understanding of client as a person, his family and
community relationships, and the nature of his problems
     B. Interpreting services and requirements to client so that he can
understand them and use them constructively
  II. Establishing helping relationships and giving appropriate initial
services to meet the need presented
     A. Being aware of and making disciplined use of own feelings
and attitudes
     B. Taking practical steps within agency functions and policy to
meet client needs on an individual basis
     C. Engaging client in examination and solution of problem by
giving respect, understanding, and acceptance
     D. Protecting client from abuse, exploitation, denial of rights, etc.,
and establishing his legal status
 III. Initiating and carrying out activities to help client function better
in his social roles and relationships
     A. Helping client to know and deal with his feeling about himself
and his relationships

---

* "Critical Requirements for Case Workers" is reprinted by permission of the
Council on Social Work Education. It was originally developed and published in
Education for Social Workers in the Public Social Services by Irving Weissman and
Mary R. Baker (New York, 1959).

B. Guiding and supporting client in carrying out plans to achieve optimum functioning or care suited to his needs

C. Arranging for services from other resources on client's behalf

D. Coordinating services to client with those of other agencies or persons

IV. Contributing to effective administrative functioning of agency

    A. Administering own work efficiently

    B. Seeking and using appropriately direction, supervision, and consultation

    C. Participating responsibly in administration of agency program and policy

V. Behaving with professional and personal self-discipline

**Critical Requirements
for Intern and
Resident Performance***

I. History

    A. Obtaining information from patient

    B. Obtaining information from other sources

    C. Using judgment

II. Physical examination

    A. Performing thorough physical examination

    B. Noting manifest signs

    C. Using appropriate technique

III. Tests and procedures

    A. Utilizing appropriate tests and procedures

    B. Applying test methods correctly

    C. Modifying tests to meet patient's needs

    D. Interpreting test results

IV. Diagnostic acumen

    A. Recognizing causes

    B. Exploring condition thoroughly

    C. Arriving at a reasonable differential diagnosis

V. Treatment

    A. Instituting the appropriate type of treatment

    B. Judging the appropriate extent of treatment

    C. Deciding on immediacy of the needs for therapy

VI. Judgment and skill in implementing care

    A. Making necessary preparations

---

* Critical Requirements for Intern and Resident Performance" is reprinted by permission of the *New England Journal of Medicine*. The list was published in an article by John P. Hubbard, M.D., *et al.* on "An Objective Evaluation of Clinical Competence." **272**:1321-1328, (June 24) 1965.

     B. Using correct methods and procedures
     C. Performing manual techniques properly
     D. Adapting method to special procedures
  VII. Continuing care
     A. Following the patient's progress
     B. Modifying treatment
     C. Planning effective follow-up care
 VIII. Physician-patient relation
     A. Establishing rapport with the patient
     B. Relieving tensions
     C. Improving patient cooperation
  IX. Responsibilities as physician
     A. For welfare of the patient
     B. For the hospital
     C. For the health of the community
     D. For the medical profession

Critical Requirements
for Orthopedic Surgeons*

    I. Skill in gathering clinical information
     A. Eliciting historical information
      1. Obtaining adequate information from the patient
      2. Consulting other physicians
      3. Checking other sources
     B. Obtaining information by physical examination
      1. Performing thorough general examination
      2. Performing relevant orthopedic checks
   II. Effectiveness in using special diagnostic methods
     A. Obtaining and interpreting x-rays
      1. Directing or ordering appropriate films
      2. Obtaining unusual, additional, or repeated films
      3. Rendering complete and adequate interpretation
     B. Obtaining additional information by other means
      1. Obtaining biopsy specimen
      2. Obtaining other laboratory data
  III. Competence in developing a diagnosis
     A. Approaching diagnosis objectively
      1. Double checking stated or referral diagnosis
      2. Persisting to establish definitive diagnosis
      3. Avoiding prejudicial analysis

* "Critical Requirements for Orthopedic Surgeons" is reprinted from a report by J. Michael Blum and Robert Fitzpatrick, *Critical Performance Requirements for Orthopedic Surgery. Part I. Method*, published by the American Institutes for Research, Pittsburgh, 1965.

B. Recognizing condition
   1. Recognizing primary disorder
   2. Recognizing underlying or associated problem

IV. Judgment in deciding on appropriate care
  A. Adapting treatment to the individual case
    1. Initiating suitable treatment for condition
    2. Treating with regard to special needs
    3. Treating with regard to age and general health
    4. Attending to contraindications
    5. Applying adequate regimen for multiple disorders
    6. Inventing, adopting, applying new techniques
  B. Determining extent and immediacy of therapy needs
    1. Choosing wisely between simple and radical approach
    2. Delaying therapy until diagnosis better established
    3. Testing milder treatment first
    4. Undertaking immediate treatment
  C. Obtaining consultation on proposed treatment
    1. Asking for opinions
    2. Incorporating suggestions

V. Judgment and skill in implementing treatment
  A. Planning the operation
    1. Reviewing literature, x-rays, other material
    2. Planning approach and procedures
  B. Making necessary preparations for operating
    1. Preparing and checking patient
    2. Readying staff, operating room, supplies
  C. Performing the operation
    1. Asking for confirmation of involved area
    2. Knowing and observing anatomic principles
    3. Using correct surgical procedures
    4. Demonstrating dexterity or skill
    5. Taking proper precautions
    6. Attending to details
    7. Persisting for maximum result
  D. Modifying operative plans according to situation
    1. Deviating from preplanned procedures
    2. Improvising with implements and materials
    3. Terminating operation when danger in continuing
  E. Handling operative complications
    1. Recognizing complications
    2. Treating complications promptly and effectively
  F. Instituting a nonoperative therapy program
    1. Using appropriate methods and devices
    2. Applying methods and devices correctly

VI. Effectiveness in treating emergency patients
   A. Handling patient
      1. Properly applying splints and other protective measures
      2. Handling and transporting carefully
   B. Performing emergency treatment
      1. Determining location and extent of injuries
      2. Attending immediately to lifesaving procedures
      3. Treating most critical needs first
      4. Obtaining and organizing help
VII. Competence in providing continuing care
   A. Paying attention postoperatively
      1. Administering suitable postoperative care
      2. Recognizing postoperative complications
      3. Adequately treating postoperative complications
   B. Monitoring patient's progress
      1. Checking on effectiveness of therapy
      2. Reassessing, altering, or repeating treatment
   C. Providing long-term care
      1. Arranging for rehabilitative care, socioeconomic assistance
      2. Explaining and monitoring home and rehabilitative care
VIII. Effectiveness of physician-patient relationship
   A. Showing concern and consideration
      1. Taking personal interest
      2. Acting in discreet, tactful, dignified manner
      3. Avoiding needless alarm, discomfort, or embarrassment
      4. Speaking honestly to patient and family
      5. Persuading patient to undertake needed care, or only needed care
   B. Relieving anxiety of patient and family
      1. Reassuring, supporting, or calming
      2. Explaining condition, treatment, prognosis, or complication
IX. Accepting responsibilities of a physician
   A. Accepting responsibility for welfare of patient
      1. Heeding the call for help
      2. Devoting necessary time and effort
      3. Meeting commitments
      4. Insisting on primacy of patient welfare
      5. Delegating responsibilities wisely
      6. Adequately supervising residents and other staff
   B. Recognizing professional capabilities and limitations
      1. Doing only what experience permits
      2. Asking for help, advice, or consultation
      3. Following instructions and advice
      4. Showing conviction and decisiveness

     5. Accepting responsibility for own errors

     6. Referring cases to other orthopedists and facilities

C. Relating effectively to other medical persons

     1. Supporting the actions of other physicians

     2. Maintaining open and honest communication

     3. Helping other physicians

     4. Relating in discreet, tactful manner

     5. Respecting other physician's responsibility to his patient

D. Displaying general medical competence

     1. Detecting, diagnosing, (treating) nonorthopedic disorders

     2. Obtaining appropriate referrals

     3. Preventing infection in hospital patients

     4. Effectively keeping and following records

E. Manifesting teaching, intellectual, and scholarly attitudes

     1. Lecturing effectively

     2. Guiding and supporting less experienced orthopedists

     3. Encouraging and contributing to fruitful discussion

     4. Contributing to medical knowledge

     5. Developing own medical knowledge and skills

F. Accepting general responsibilities to profession and community

     1. Serving the profession

     2. Serving the community

     3. Maintaining personal and intellectual integrity

Appendix II

Expected Student Behavior

in Selected

Clinical Areas

(BASED ON COURSE OBJECTIVES)

I. Nursing Care of Patients with Gynecologic Conditions
II. Nursing Care of Patients in the Recovery Room
III. Nursing Care of Patients in the Outpatient Department
IV. Team Relationships

These expected behaviors have been designed for selected clinical areas. They are not intended to be used in every nursing situation. Each nursing program should design its own for its specific use depending on the course objectives. They are intended to be used as guides upon which to construct lists of expected behaviors appropriate for other nursing situations.

I. Course in Nursing Care of Patients
with Gynecologic Conditions

A student who meets the objectives of this course in both theory and planned clinical experience will be expected to do the following:

1. Identify and use special terminology to describe gynecologic conditions.
2. Apply skills of observation recording pertinent facts.
3. Utilize concepts of nursing care learned previous to the gynecologic experience.
4. Establish rapport with patient and inspire confidence.
5. Identify the psychologic problems that occur as a result of mechanical disturbances or removal of organs in the female.
6. Teach individual patients and/or their families in relation to expected symptoms and responses of those having gynecologic disorders.

7. Prepare patient for diagnostic tests and procedures such as:
   a. Pelvic examination
   b. Vaginal smear
   c. Vaginal douche
8. Convey understanding in relation to psychologic and physical trauma.
9. Listen to patients. Know when to react.
10. Prevent unnecessary exposure.
11. Respect the patient's right to privacy.
12. Know how to fill out requisitions for tests and specimens.
13. Shave preparation for surgery.
14. Be familiar with the names and types of instruments used in the examination of gynecologic patients.
15. Drape patient and assist with pelvic and breast examinations.
16. Assist with preparation of smears.
17. Save all tissues and clots from bleeding patients and preserve for examination.
18. Know how to prepare previable products of conception.
19. Record accurately.
20. Report promptly pertinent information to proper source.
21. Check vital signs as patient's condition indicates. Record.
22. Know action, dosage, and precautions of medications used in the medical care plan.
23. Take precautionary measures in caring for patients with venereal disease.
24. Prepare a nursing care plan consistent with the medical care plan for a patient with:
    a. Postoperative hysterectomy
    b. Radium insertion (vaginal)
    c. Postoperative breast surgery.
25. Check voiding after Foley catheter is removed.
26. Prepare patient for radium insertion procedure.
27. Take precautions for caring for a patient with radium:
    a. Bed signs
    b. Exposure time
    c. Linen check
28. Discuss emergency actions necessary in case of accidents.
29. Identify radiation sickness.
30. Assist the physician with removal of radium.
31. Describe care following removal of radium.
32. Describe care of skin with radiation burns.
33. Instruct patients in self-examination of the breast.
34. Prepare patient psychologically and physically for breast surgery.
35. Be alert to psychologic needs.

36. Observe operative area and report signs of infection (observe skin closely for radiation burns if used).
37. Encourage patients to void postoperatively.
38. Teach and have patient return demonstration of postoperative arm exercises following mastectomy.
39. Describe method used to make temporary breast prosthesis.
40. Suggest fitting by a corsetiere for various types of breast prosthesis.
41. Inform patient and families of:
    a. Referral system
    b. Early examination and treatment
    c. American Cancer Society services
    d. Seven danger signals of cancer
42. Plan a course of action for home care. Discuss rehabilitation plans with patient and/or family.

II. Unit on Nursing Care of Patients
in the Recovery Room

A student who meets the objectives of this unit in both theory and planned clinical experience will be expected to do the following:

1. Note, report, and record significant changes in cardinal symptoms of postoperative patients.
2. Observe and chart every 15 minutes:
    a. Blood pressure
    b. Pulse rate, rhythm, and volume
    c. Respirations—rate, rhythm, and volume
    d. Condition and color of the skin
    e. Level of consciousness and changes in the level of consciousness
    f. Presence of drains, drainage tubing, or catheters
3. Maintain a patent airway.
4. Identify and report signs of postoperative complaints, discomforts, and complications such as:
    a. Pain
    b. Restlessness and apprehension
    c. Respiratory complications including obstruction, laryngospasm, aspiration, and atelectasis.
    d. Shock
    e. Circulatory impairment and complications such as hemorrhage, thrombosis, and cardiac arrest
    f. Vomiting and abdominal distention
    g. Urinary retention and overflow
    h. Wound dehiscence
    i. Abnormal drainage
5. Demonstrate and operate the following equipment and discuss the procedures associated with its use:

    a. Oxygen apparatus

    b. Suction machines

    c. Resuscitator

6. List the location of and indications for use of following:
    a. Cardiac arrest trays
    b. Venesection trays
    c. Emergency drugs
    d. Routine drugs
    e. Tracheotomy trays
7. Describe the proper position for various types of surgery.
8. Protect the patient during the restless phase with pillows or padding.
9. Exercise and use proper restraints.
10. Withhold all oral fluids unless ordered.
11. Measure and record intake and output on patients with Levin tubes and other types of drainage tubing and on all patients where intake and output are specifically ordered.
12. Check for infiltration of intravenous solutions, proper rate of flow and proper position and circulation of extremity.
13. Demonstrate proper method of lifting, moving, turning, and transporting the patient.
14. Demonstrate proper technique for arousing a patient.
15. Describe and demonstrate proper connection of drains for:
    a. Thoracotomy
    b. Suction machines
    c. Levin tubes
    d. Catheters
16. Describe the stages of anesthesia.
17. Discuss the effects of the various anesthetics and identify reactions in each type.
18. Ensure patient safety and comfort.
19. Respect the patient's right to privacy.
    a. Prevent unnecessary exposure.
    b. Hold in confidence any information divulged by patient while reacting from anesthesia.
    c. Avoid unnecessary conversation about the patient's condition at the bedside.
    d. Hold in confidence information found on the chart and do not divulge to the patient or his family.
20. Recognize that the last sense lost before anesthesia and the first one regained after anesthesia is hearing.
21. Change position frequently to prevent postoperative complications and pressure areas unless otherwise ordered.
22. Differentiate between physical and psychologic needs of the patient in relation to his requests.

23. Refer all inquiries (telephone or otherwise) concerning the patient to the graduate nurse.
24. Maintain composure in emergency situations.
25. Establish and maintain good interpersonal relationships with recovery room personnel for more effective patient care.
26. Report condition of patient periodically to charge nurse.
27. Be alert to and responsible for the total care of the patient, including physical, psychologic, and environmental aspects.
28. Locate and demonstrate use of fire extinguishers.

III. Unit on Nursing Care of Patients in the Outpatient Department

A student who meets the objectives of this unit in both theory and planned clinical experience will be expected to do the following:

1. Describe the outpatient department as a community service for the care of the ambulatory patient who is in need of medical supervision.
2. Discuss the outpatient department services available to members of the community through special programs such as periodical mass surveys for glaucoma and immunization against poliomyelitis.
3. Implement the policies of the outpatient department and the various clinics.
4. Discuss the routines for an admission of a patient to the hospital through the outpatient department.
5. Participate in all clinics, rendering safe patient care.
   a. Know the routines of the different clinics.
   b. Know the responsibilities of the nurse in each clinic.
   c. Know how to prepare patients for all clinics.
   d. Report unusual symptoms to the nurse in charge of the clinic.
   e. Carry out specific procedures as taught, always considering the safety and dignity of the patient.
6. Locate supplies for the different clinics.
7. Locate and demonstrate how to operate fire extinguishers.
8. Locate exits in outpatient department.
9. Discuss need for and carry out emergency measures when necessary.
10. Interview and teach the patient and/or member of the family.
    a. Identify and meet, as nearly as possible, the psychologic needs of the patient and family.
    b. Identify the relationship of the socioeconomic needs of the patient to total patient care.
    c. Identify and meet, through referral to the medical social worker or other community agencies, the socioeconomic and nursing needs of the patient.
    d. Identify and meet the need to reinforce the physician's orders.

e. Instruct the patients and/or member of the family in specific health measures, general health hygiene, and various procedures as indicated.

f. Teach procedures with adaptation to home facilities.

11. Complete Department of Public Assistance prescription blanks after the physician has written and signed them.

12. Initiate requisitions, as ordered, in each clinic.

13. Discuss the importance of care in preserving and preparing laboratory specimens.

14. Notify the clerk of diagnostic tests ordered for the patient.

15. Understand the role of the nursing service office and auxiliary personnel.

16. Function in a calm, pleasant manner to provide better patient care and smooth operation of the outpatient department.

IV. Unit on Team Relationships

A student who meets the objectives of this unit in both theory and planned clinical experience will be expected to do the following:

1. Discuss the purpose of organizational charts, and be able to follow lines of authority as defined in them.

2. Identify the need for responsibility being definitely centralized.

3. List the objectives of nursing service department and uphold the standards.

4. Describe the place of the head nurse in the nursing service structure and the scope of her responsibilities.

5. Attend a nursing service organization meeting and identify value of same.

6. List the necessary qualifications and limitations of the following personnel:
   a. Licensed practical nurse
   b. Nurse's aide
   c. Orderly
   d. Ward secretary
   e. Inhalation therapist

7. List the objectives and policies of the Inservice Education program.

8. Attend representative programs of the Inservice Education Department.

9. Describe the functions and responsibilities of various members of the team.

10. Assist the head nurse in implementing hospital policies and procedures.

11. Assist the head nurse in identifying and providing care to meet the needs of the individual patients.

12. Safeguard patients from injury by keeping equipment in good order.
13. Make rounds routinely to make certain patient needs are being met.
14. Assume delegated responsibility without undue stress, meet daily activities with more confidence, and become more self-directive.
15. Interpret and note physician's orders.
16. Assist in promoting relationships that will ensure mutual cooperation and support not only within the unit but between departments in the hospital.
17. Identify, analyze, and solve problems with the assistance of the head nurse.
18. Anticipate possible emergencies and meet them intelligently.
19. Assist in maintaining open lines of communication.
20. Assist the head nurse in planning weekly schedules for all personnel.
21. Demonstrate how to calculate nursing hours per patient.
22. Assist in planning daily team assignments, giving consideration to individual patients as well as the abilities and satisfaction of the personnel.
23. Assist in developing nursing care plans.
24. Assume responsibility under direction for ordering linens, supplies, and equipment.
25. Assist the head nurse in orienting new personnel according to their needs and level of experience using the floor orientation guide.
26. Review the unit budget with the head nurse.
27. Assume greater responsibility for conserving time, effort, and materials.
28. Apply the principles of leadership and assist in directing the work of auxiliary personnel.
29. Assist the head nurse in evaluating personnel and observe the value of recording critical incidents.
30. Record, give reports, and write reports with clarity and accuracy.
31. Assist in maintaining all records according to hospital procedures and standards.

Appendix III
Performance
Descriptions*

I. Taking temperature
  Oral temperature
  Rectal temperature
  Axillary temperature
II. Taking pulse
III. Counting respiration

I–A. Taking Temperature—Oral
TASK: Takes patient's temperature. Subtask 1: Takes oral temperature.
JOB TITLE: Nurse.
OBJECT ACTED UPON: Patient.
INFORMATION GUIDING ACTION: Recall, nursing or doctor's order, nursing procedure book.
TOOLS: Equipment tray, jar of soap and water, jar of clear water, tissues, oral thermometer, container for waste, dish of disinfectant (usually 70% alcohol), temperature sheet or note paper for recording temperature.
ACTION: Executes a procedure.

1. Assists the patient to assume a sitting or lying position. (Temperatures are not taken while patient is standing or walking about because of the danger of breakage of thermometer.)
2. Examines the thermometer for chips or breaks.

* The Performance Descriptions listed in this Appendix and those in the earlier section of the book were developed by Mrs. Angeline Marchese Jacobs, R.N., in connection with a project on vocational education conducted by the American Institutes for Research under a grant from the Ford Foundation.

3. Examines thermometer to ensure mercury is below 35° C. or 90° F. If not, shakes thermometer down with a quick downward and outward movement of the wrist.

Precaution: Must be careful that hand or thermometer does not hit against anything.

Note: Some hospitals use Clay-Adams thermometer holders with automatic shake-down characteristics.

4. Ascertains whether patient has just had a hot or cold drink. If he has, waits 15 minutes to take temperature.
5. Places bulb of thermometer under patient's tongue (to ensure proximity to large blood vessels).
6. Instructs patient to hold tongue down and to keep mouth closed while thermometer is in place for three minutes (to allow the air in the mouth to warm to body temperature).

Precautions: Usually nurse should stay with patient the entire three minutes to prevent possible accidents and to ensure reliability of the temperature measurement. The nurse should exercise her own judgment as to whether the patient's condition and integrity warrant leaving him alone. The nurse utilizes the three minutes to count the pulse and respiration.

7. Removes the thermometer from patient's mouth.
8. Wipes thermometer with tissue or cotton ball soaked with soap and water. Wipes with a firm, rotary motion toward the bulb to remove the mucus from the thermometer before it dries.

Note: Mucus is very difficult to remove when dry and, in chemical disinfection, prevents adequate disinfecting by providing protection to the microorganisms.

9. Discards tissue in waste containers.
10. Holds thermometer in horizontal position at eye level and rotates to make bar of mercury visible. Holds thermometer at tip to avoid touching portion that has been in patient's mouth and thus prevent spread of microorganisms to other patients.
11. Reads degree of temperature from scale. (Scale range is usually 92–110° F. or 33°–43° C.)
12. Rinses soap from thermometer with tissue moistened in clear water (to prevent chemical action of soap and disinfectant, which may hinder disinfecting).
13. Places thermometer in disinfectant solution for prescribed time. (Fifteen minutes is usual, but this varies with the disinfectant.)

Note: Thermometer should be disinfected whether it is to be used for another patient (to prevent cross-infection) or for the same patient (to prevent autoreinfection). Alcohol is usually used as it has a specific action on many dangerous mouth organisms, such as the tubercle bacillus.

14. Notes temperature reading on temperature sheet or note paper, identifies patient adequately.
15. Later, transcribes temperature recording to graphic record.
16. If temperature is extraordinarily high (or low), reports this to the charge nurse or doctor immediately, in addition to recording it on the chart. These critical temperatures vary among institutions, but are usually above 101° F. (38° C.) or below 96° F. (36° C.)

Contingencies:
1. If a thermometer is broken while in a patient's mouth (or anus or axilla), nurse removes all particles of glass and notifies charge nurse and/or physician at once.
2. When oral temperature is contraindicated, rectal or axillary temperature is taken, depending on patient's condition. Contraindications for oral temperature are:
   a. Uncooperative patient
   b. Patient in oxygen tent
   c. Oral or nasal surgery
   d. Nasal obstruction
   e. Dyspnea or acute respiratory distress
   f. Acute coughing
   g. Dry, inflamed mouth
   h. Unconscious or delirious patient
   i. Very young patient

General note: Taking temperature is a repetitive task. The usual patient has his temperature taken once in the morning and once in the evening. More frequent readings (every four hours) are required in the following instances:

   a. All postoperative patients for a certain period postoperatively, usually 24 to 48 hours.
   b. All seriously ill patients.
   c. Patients who have had an elevated temperature—usually until temperature returns to normal.

Even more frequent temperature readings (every hour) may be ordered by the doctor for some patients with special surgery, with very high fevers, or with chills.

COMPLETION INDICATOR: Temperature recorded on patient's chart.

I–B. Taking Temperature—Rectal

JOB TITLE: Nurse.

TASK: Takes patient's temperature. Subtask 2: Takes rectal temperature.

OBJECT ACTED UPON: Patient.

INFORMATION GUIDING ACTION: Recall, nursing orders, doctor's orders, nursing procedure book.

TOOLS: Rectal thermometer, equipment tray, lubricant, tissues, waste container, temperature sheet or note paper, container of soap and water, clear water, container of disinfectant.

ACTION: Executes a procedure.

1. Explains to patient why rectal temperature is necessary (if indicated).
2. Ensures that thermometer is a rectal thermometer (rounded bulb rather than long tapered one). Usually the hospital labels rectal thermometers with such devices as a red-painted tip.
3. Assists patient to assume Sims's position unless contraindicated (patient on side, lower leg extended, upper leg flexed and drawn up close to abdomen).

Note: If Sims's position is contraindicated, allows patient to lie on back and bring up knees slightly with legs apart.

4. In either case, drapes patient to avoid embarrassment.
5. Ensures thermometer reads below 35° C.
6. Squeezes small amount of lubricant (usually water-soluble lubricant) on tissue and lubricates thermometer.
7. Discards tissue into waste container.
8. Separates buttocks to expose anus clearly.

Precautions: Attempting to insert thermometer without clear view of the opening may result in injury to the patient.

9. Inserts thermometer slowly past sphincter muscle, leaving about one-half of the thermometer visible.
10. Holds thermometer in place a minimum of two minutes.

Precaution: Thermometer should always be held in place, but this is especially important for very sick, delirious, very young, or uncooperative patients.

11. Removes thermometer and wipes with a soaped tissue with a rotary motion toward the bulb. Discards tissue.
12. Reads thermometer.
13. Cleans thermometer.
14. Records temperature reading.

Contingencies:
1. Rectal temperatures are taken when oral temperatures are contraindicated. Rectal temperatures, however, may also be contraindicated—usually because of rectal obstruction, hemorrhoids or other disorders, or rectal surgery. In such a case, axillary temperature should be taken.
2. If thermometer breaks while in patient's anus, glass should be removed immediately, and charge nurse and/or doctor notified.

Safety Precautions:
1. Thermometer must be well lubricated to prevent irritation.
2. Thermometer must not be inserted too far.
3. Thermometer should always be held in place the full two minutes.

COMPLETION INDICATOR: Temperature has been recorded on patient's chart.

I–C. Taking Temperature—Axillary

JOB TITLE: Nurse.

TASK: Takes patient's temperature. Subtask 3: Takes axillary temperature.

OBJECT ACTED UPON: Patient.

INFORMATION GUIDING ACTION: Recall, nursing or doctor's order, nursing procedure book.

TOOLS: Same equipment as for oral temperature plus bath towel.

ACTION: Executes a procedure.

1. Explains to patient why axillary temperature is necessary (if indicated).
2. Removes gown from shoulder, being careful not to expose patient.
3. Wipes axilla dry with bath towel.
4. Ensures mercury is below 35° C.
5. Places bulb of thermometer in hollow of axilla with stem protruding toward the chest.
6. Places arm across chest (asks patient to grasp opposite shoulder). This keeps thermometer in place.
7. Leaves thermometer in place for ten minutes. Uses judgment as to whether patient may be left alone for this much time.
8. Proceeds as with oral temperature.

Note: Axillary temperatures are taken when both oral and rectal temperatures are contraindicated. It usually is less accurate than other methods of temperature measurement, therefore should be taken only when absolutely necessary. Usually permission of the charge nurse is required. If the practical nurse is the charge nurse, she must exercise proper judgment in this regard.

Contingencies:
1. The armpit must be dry, and the thermometer so placed that it will not touch the clothing or be exposed to the air.
2. When patient is unable to put her hand on shoulder herself, the nurse must help her to do so.
3. When taking a child's axillary temperature, holds the thermometer in place the entire time.
4. Method is not used if patient is so thin that there is a hollow under the arm which would make it impossible to provide an air-tight environment. If this is true, and both oral and rectal temperatures are clearly contraindicated, the doctor should be consulted as to the best method to be used.
5. In case of breakage, the glass is removed from the axilla and the charge nurse and/or doctor are notified immediately.

COMPLETION INDICATOR: Temperature recorded on patient's chart.

II. Taking Pulse

JOB TITLE: Nurse.
TASK: Takes patient's pulse.
OBJECT ACTED UPON: Patient.
INFORMATION GUIDING ACTION: Recall, nursing or doctor's orders.
TOOLS: Timepiece with second hand, pad and pencil.
ACTION: Executes a procedure.
1. Assists patient to sitting or lying position (pulse is less stable when patient is standing or walking).
2. Places extremity, well supported, in a comfortable position.
3. Locates pulse with fingertips (does not use thumb, which has its own artery and thus might obscure patient's pulse). Compresses artery against underlying bone, adjusting pressure of fingertips as necessary. Usually the radial artery on the wrist is used.

Contingencies: If for some reason the radial artery cannot be used, the pulse beat can be obtained (by the same method) from—
    a. Temporal artery on the side of the forehead
    b. Carotid artery in the neck
    c. Femoral artery in the groin
    d. Popliteal artery (back of knee)
    e. Tibial artery (leg)

If pulse must be taken in an area other than the radial artery, the nurse should explain the reason to the patient in such a way as to be reassuring.
4. Counts the beats in a given time period. Sixty seconds is preferable as it gives the nurse an opportunity to note irregularities of rhythm

which might not be detectable in a shorter period.

5. Notes any irregularities of rhythm, intensity, or strength of the pulse. If any irregularities are noted, recounts pulse at least one full minute.
6. Notes pulse rate and character on TPR sheet or note paper, properly identified, so it will not be forgotten.
7. Transcribes pulse rate to graphic chart. Notes any irregularities in appropriate place on chart.
8. Reports any serious irregularities immediately to charge nurse or doctor. These include (1) excessively slow rate (below 50 per minute). This is important in cardiac patients, especially those on digitalis, where a heart rate of below 40 per minute may be a contraindication to giving the patient his medication. (2) Excessively fast rate (above 100 per minute). This is often an indication of hemorrhage in postoperative patients or of distress in a cardiac patient. (3) Irregularities of rhythm (important in postoperative and cardiac patients).

Contingencies: Pulse should not be counted after patient has had a painful physical or emotional experience or has been exercising.

General Note: Pulse is taken twice a day on the usual patient. It is ordered more frequently when indicated by the patient's condition. (See same indications under taking temperature.) Pulse may be ordered every five minutes following some treatments or surgery.

COMPLETION INDICATOR: Pulse rate and character are properly recorded on chart.

III. Counting Respiration
JOB TITLE: Nurse
TASK: Counts patient's respiration.
OBJECT ACTED UPON: Patient.
INFORMATION GUIDING ACTION: Recall, nursing or doctor's order.
TOOLS: Watch with second hand, pad and pencil.
ACTION: Executes a procedure.

1. When taking pulse, either before or after counting (see Task II), watches the respirations and counts them by looking at the chest as it rises and falls.
2. Counts number of respirations per minute; usually counts for one full minute.
3. Notes irregularities in breathing (too rapid—above 20 per minute; too slow—below 12 per minute) dyspnea, apnea, other difficulties.
4. Reports irregularities to charge nurse and/or doctor immediately.

5. Notes respiration rate and character with patient's name on TPR sheet or note paper.
6. Transcribes respiration rate to graphic record. Notes irregularities in appropriate place on chart.

Precautions: Task is performed so that patient will think that it is the pulse beat being recorded. Calling attention to the fact that one is taking a respiration count will probably make the patient breathe unnaturally. Respirations should not be counted immediately after the patient has exercised, become excited, or had extreme physical pain.

COMPLETION INDICATOR: Patient's respiration rate and character are recorded properly.

Index

225